Susan M. Enguídanos, MPH, PhD
Editor

Evidence-Based Interventions for Community Dwelling Older Adults

Evidence-Based Interventions for Community Dwelling Older Adults has been co-published simultaneously as *Home Health Care Services Quarterly*, Volume 25, Numbers 1/2 2006.

*Pre-publication
REVIEWS,
COMMENTARIES,
EVALUATIONS . . .*

"The practice of medicine has to change to meet the challenge of our growing senior population. This collection of papers exemplifies the evolution of medical care from tacit knowledge to evidence-based. By covering critical issues of medications, falls, palliative care, depression and targeting of social services, these significant translational research papers provide a framework for implementation by health care practitioners. As a physician, I find this collection to be EXTREMELY VALUABLE in providing justification and an action plan for change to better care for our seniors."

Karen Lynn Josephson, MD
*Geriatrician for Health Care Partners
Voluntary Faculty
USC Keck School of Medicine*

Evidence-Based Interventions for Community Dwelling Older Adults

Evidence-Based Interventions for Community Dwelling Older Adults has been co-published simultaneously as *Home Health Care Services Quarterly*, Volume 25, Numbers 1/2 2006.

Monographic Separates from *Home Health Care Services Quarterly*™

For additional information on these and other Haworth Press titles, including descriptions, tables of contents, reviews, and prices, use the QuickSearch catalog at http://www.HaworthPress.com.

Evidence-Based Interventions for Community Dwelling Older Adults, edited by Susan M. Enguídanos, MPH, PhD (Vol. 25, No. 1/2, 2006). *An overview of evidence-based programs that can improve the health of seniors living in community-based settings.*

Improving Medication Management in Home Care: Issues and Solutions, edited by Dennee Frey, PharmD (Vol. 24, No. 1/2, 2005). *A comprehensive examination of the issues and challenges faced in preventing medication errors with effective strategies for managing medication use in home and community care settings.*

A New Look at Community-Based Respite Programs: Utilization, Satisfaction, and Development, edited by Rhonda J.V. Montgomery, PhD (Vol. 21, No. 3/4, 2002). *"Clear, straightforward, and well focused on practical issues of service delivery . . . maintains a high standard of scholarship. A must-read for anyone interested in planning or evaluating respite services . . . . The first large-scale, longitudinal study of respite use. Service professionals, policymakers, and researchers in health policy, gerontology, and medical sociology will find the text of great value." (Judith G. Gonyea, PhD, Associate Professor, Boston University School of Social Work)*

The Next Generation of AIDS Patients: Service Needs and Vulnerabilities, edited by George J. Huba, PhD, Lisa A. Melchoir, PhD, A. T. Panter, PhD, Vivian B. Brown, PhD, David A. Cherin, PhD, and June Simmons, LCSW (Vol. 19, No. 1/2, 2001). *"Especially interesting in this volume is the presentation of an empirical model (CHAID) that both community-based organizations and service delivery systems can use to analyze client input to monitor and refine their HIV services." (Donna G. Anderson, PhD, MPH, Associate Professor, University of Colorado Health Sciences Center)*

AIDS Capitation, edited by David Alex Cherin, PhD, and G. J. Huba, PhD (Vol. 17, No. 1, 1998). *"A valuable resource to those interested in the blending of curative and palliative care and the application of this blended approach to catastrophic disease management." (Victor L. Kovner, MD, FACP, Medical Director, Sun Alliance Hospice)*

Personal Response Systems: An International Report of a New Home Care Service, edited by Andrew S. Dibner, PhD (Vol. 13, No. 3/4, 1993). *"Does a great service by reporting the forward strides taking place in other nations in the use of personal response systems (PRS)." (Daniel Thursz, DSW, ACSW, President, The National Council of Aging, Inc., Washington, DC)*

Facilitating Self Care Practices in the Elderly, edited by Barbara J. Horn, PhD, RN (Vol. 11, No. 1/2, 1990). *"Useful to researchers, practitioners, caregivers, and agencies providing care services to the elderly ill at home." (The Indian Journal of Social Work)*

Quality Impact of Home Care for the Elderly, edited by Francis G. Caro, PhD, and Arthur E. Blank, PhD (Vol. 9, No. 2/3, 1989). *"An excellent source of information for those wishing to increase their understanding of the home health care system or improve its effectiveness in their own community." (American Journal of Occupational Therapy)*

Worlds Apart?: Long-Term Care in Australia and the United States, edited by Sandra J. Newman, PhD (Vol. 8, No. 3, 1988). *An insightful comparison of how Australia and the United States are responding to the long-term care needs of the elderly.*

Health Care for the Elderly: Regional Responses for National Policy Issues, edited by Kathleen Gainor Andreoli, DSN, Leigh Anne Musser, MPH, and Stanley Joel Reiser, MD, PhD (Vol. 7, No. 3/4, 1987). *"One of the best, most comprehensive, and most penetratingly analytical works on elderly health care now available." (Health and Social Work)*

International Perspectives on Long-Term Care, edited by Laura Reif and Brahna Trager (Vol. 5, No. 3/4, 1985). *Experts from around the world address organizational and cost issues while offering innovative solutions for common problems in long-term care.*

Community-Based Systems of Long-Term Care, edited by Rick T. Zawadski, PhD (Vol. 4, No. 3/4, 1984). *Essential information on planning long-term health care services for the community.*

The Chronically Limited Elderly: The Case for a National Policy for In-Home and Supportive Community-Based Services, edited by Howard A. Palley, PhD, and Julianne S. Oktay, PhD (Vol. 4, No. 2, 1983). *"Compelling reading for those concerned about the non-institutional care of impaired elderly persons." (The Gerontologist)*

Family Home Care: Critical Issues for Services and Policies, edited by Robert Perlman, PhD (Vol. 3, No. 3/4, 1983). *"An important reference for those professionals working in the field of home health care." (Contemporary Sociology)*

Home Health Care and National Health Policy, edited by Brahna Trager (Vol. 1, No. 2, 1980). *A concise study of the current status of home health care in the United States.*

Evidence-Based Interventions for Community Dwelling Older Adults

Susan M. Enguídanos, MPH, PhD
Editor

Evidence-Based Interventions for Community Dwelling Older Adults has been co-published simultaneously as *Home Health Care Services Quarterly*, Volume 25, Numbers 1/2 2006.

The Haworth Press, Inc.

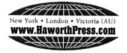

New York • London • Victoria (AU)
www.HaworthPress.com

Evidence-Based Interventions for Community Dwelling Older Adults has been co-published simultaneously as *Home Health Care Services Quarterly*™, Volume 25, Numbers 1/2 2006.

The development, preparation, and publication of this work has been undertaken with great care. However, the publisher, employees, editors, and agents of The Haworth Press and all imprints of The Haworth Press, Inc., including The Haworth Medical Press® and Pharmaceutical Products Press®, are not responsible for any errors contained herein or for consequences that may ensue from use of materials or information contained in this work. With regard to case studies, identities and circumstances of individuals discussed herein have been changed to protect confidentiality. Any resemblance to actual persons, living or dead, is entirely coincidental.

The Haworth Press is committed to the dissemination of ideas and information according to the highest standards of intellectual freedom and the free exchange of ideas. Statements made and opinions expressed in this publication do not necessarily reflect the views of the Publisher, Directors, management, or staff of The Haworth Press, Inc., or an endorsement by them.

Cover design by Lora Wiggins

Library of Congress Cataloging-in-Publication Data

Evidence-based interventions for community dwelling older adults / Susan M. Enguídanos, editor.
    p. cm.
    "Co-published simultaneously as Home Health care Servcices Quarterly, Volume 25, Numbers 1/2 2006."
    Includes bibliographical references and index.
    ISBN-13: 978-0-7890-3283-6 (hard cover : alk. paper)
    ISBN-10: 0-7890-3283-X (hard cover : alk. paper)
    ISBN-13: 978-0-7890-3284-3 (soft cover : alk. paper)
    ISBN-10: 0-7890-3284-8 (soft cover : alk. paper)
    1. Community health services for older people. 2. Evidence-based medicine. 3. Older people–Services for. 4. Older people–Care. I. Enguídanos, Susan M. II. Home health care services quarterly.
RA564.8.E95 2006
362.198'97–dc22   2005035757

Indexing, Abstracting & Website/Internet Coverage

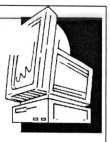

This section provides you with a list of major indexing & abstracting services and other tools for bibliographic access. That is to say, each service began covering this periodical during the year noted in the right column. Most Websites which are listed below have indicated that they will either post, disseminate, compile, archive, cite or alert their own Website users with research-based content from this work. (This list is as current as the copyright date of this publication.)

(continued)

(continued)

  * Exact start date to come

(continued)

Special Bibliographic Notes related to special journal issues
(separates) and indexing/abstracting:

- indexing/abstracting services in this list will also cover material in any "separate" that is co-published simultaneously with Haworth's special thematic journal issue or DocuSerial. Indexing/abstracting usually covers material at the article/chapter level.
- monographic co-editions are intended for either non-subscribers or libraries which intend to purchase a second copy for their circulating collections.
- monographic co-editions are reported to all jobbers/wholesalers/approval plans. The source journal is listed as the "series" to assist the prevention of duplicate purchasing in the same manner utilized for books-in-series.
- to facilitate user/access services all indexing/abstracting services are encouraged to utilize the co-indexing entry note indicated at the bottom of the first page of each article/chapter/contribution.
- this is intended to assist a library user of any reference tool (whether print, electronic, online, or CD-ROM) to locate the monographic version if the library has purchased this version but not a subscription to the source journal.
- individual articles/chapters in any Haworth publication are also available through the Haworth Document Delivery Service (HDDS).

Evidence-Based Interventions for Community Dwelling Older Adults

CONTENTS

ABOUT THE EDITOR

Susan Enguídanos, MPH, PhD, has a multidisciplinary background evident in her educational and professional history. She obtained her BA in Psychology at UCLA, Master's degree in Public Health at California State University, Long Beach, and her doctorate degree in Social Work at USC. She has more than 12 years of experience conducting research on an array of topics ranging from developing community-based HIV/AIDS prevention programs to identifying statewide ethnic disparities in access to end-of-life care. Her areas of research currently focus on geriatric health and end of life care issues, with specific projects in the area of geriatric care management, physician-patient communications, and new models of end-of-life care. Further she has special interest in investigating barriers and facilitators associated with implementing evidence-based models in social work practice within medical and community-based settings. Dr. Enguídanos is currently co-Principal Investigator on a project entitled "Integrating Depression Care into Geriatric Care Management," a two-year study testing the efficacy of a multifaceted model of depression care integrated into care management practices. She is also co-Principal Investigator of a study investigating an evidence-based social work intervention in primary care. She serves as the evaluator on several other projects, including a medications management program for older adults, a project on naturally occurring retirement communities, a needs assessment identifying the psychosocial service needs of people with Parkinson's disease, and a program aimed at improving the health of the elderly with multiple chronic diseases. She has published the findings from her research in several peer-reviewed journals including *Journal of American Geriatric Society, Journal of Social Work in End of Life & Palliative Care, Social Work in Health Care, Journal of Palliative Medicine*, and *Drugs in Society*. She is an active member of Gerontological Society of America and American Society of Aging and has presented results of her work at many of these and other professional meetings and conferences. Further, her research on an end of life care model received a national Kaiser Permanente Award for quality and has been replicated in Kaiser's throughout Southern California. The impact of Dr. Enguídanos' research has been far reaching, resulting in the development of programs that are improving the delivery of healthcare nationally for people at the end-life-life and the elderly.

Foreword

In 2005, the editor of a leading health journal proclaimed that after fifteen years, evidence-based medicine "has arrived in full flower."[1] The journal devoted an issue to an in-depth state-of-the-science examination of evidence-based medicine's past, present and future. Notably absent from this collection of articles was any explicit mention of the role of individual patients, family caregivers, home health care service agencies, or community based organizations.

The United States' health care delivery system has embraced evidence-based medicine, largely based on its potential to reduce unwanted variation and reign in on escalating health care costs. We must recognize, however, that evidence-based medicine is largely a recycling of core public health principles as they relate to population-based care and optimal use of limited resources. Early on, evidence-based medicine primarily focused on supporting physician decision-making, reinforcing the paradigm of a one-way flow of advice and information from doctor to patient; which has become increasingly less relevant to an era where chronic illness and its accompanying need for self-management support dominate the health care landscape. What followed were attempts to construct clinical guidelines designed to reduce variation and inform insurance coverage decisions whereby the patient was relegated the role of passive recipient and the context or environment in which their chronic conditions were experienced was by and large ignored. Looking to the future, if we truly want to improve health care outcomes, we need to expand our approaches beyond the traditional conception of evidence-based medicine to engaging patients and their family caregivers in health promotion and chronic illness self-management in their

---

[Haworth co-indexing entry note]: "Foreword." Coleman, Eric A., and Nancy Gibbs. Co-published simultaneously in *Home Health Care Services Quarterly* (The Haworth Press, Inc.) Vol. 25, No. 1/2, 2006, pp. xix-xxi; and: *Evidence-Based Interventions for Community Dwelling Older Adults* (ed: Susan M. Enguídanos) The Haworth Press, Inc., 2006, pp. xv-xvii. Single or multiple copies of this article are available for a fee from The Haworth Document Delivery Service [1-800-HAWORTH, 9:00 a.m. - 5:00 p.m. (EST). E-mail address: docdelivery@haworthpress.com].

homes and in their communities. We must also appreciate the fact that patient-centered care may require allowance for some desired variation.

It is for these very reasons that this volume represents a critical milestone in the evolution of evidence-based medicine. The articles that comprise this special collection contribute to the broader evidence-base of how to more effectively manage care beyond the hospital or clinic; expanding into home and community settings. The authors of these models present compelling evidence for their effectiveness with respect to prevention and treatment. By addressing the core elements of health promotion and high quality care for older adults including physical activity, falls prevention, medication management, strategies to reduce depression, and palliative care, these authors ultimately bring the efforts and experience of community-based aging service providers and clinic-based providers closer together to improve outcomes for older adults. Once more, these articles highlight the invaluable contributions of social workers, pharmacists, and care managers. Finally, collectively these articles also illustrate the importance of leadership in extending evidence-based medicine to community-based settings, through the efforts of the Administration on Aging, National Council on Aging, and the Centers for Disease Control. The resulting evidence of success of these models will undoubtedly facilitate further adoption into other communities and perhaps also instruct on how to optimally allocate scarce resources. I hope you will join me in this excitement and read forward with enthusiasm.

Eric A. Coleman, MD, MPH
Associate Professor
Divisions of Health Care Policy and Research and Geriatric Medicine
University of Colorado Health Sciences Center

NOTE

1. Health Affairs 2005:24(1):7

As a primary care physician and later as a geriatrician practicing in the world of home and long term care, I greatly appreciate the evolution of practice from 'community standard' and 'usual and customary' to evidenced-based. I was introduced to the concept of evidenced-based medicine by Dr. David Eddy in his visionary leadership of my medical group. We were all skeptical. How could we change what we believed was individualized, appropriate care into a standardized approach? Wouldn't that be cookbook medicine? Now in 2005, I congratulate the authors of this edition who contribute to clinical and community-based practice through their discussion of existing evidenced based programs as well as the barriers that are faced in embracing these programs. This work covers very important areas of clinical practice for chronically ill and older adults.

In geriatrics, a relatively new specialty in American medicine, our knowledge of how to appropriately care for older adults has evolved over the past 25 years. For years we in geriatrics have preached about geriatric syndromes such as falls, depression, and polypharmacy that are very significant, but whose clinical impact is under recognized in older patients. We have promoted care management as a mechanism to assist our frail and chronically ill patients to negotiate complex health care systems and their own health problems without a clear understanding about what components of care management work and don't work. We have promoted the need for older patients to engage in physical activity and to have access to quality palliative and end of life care because it is 'the right thing to do' and yet, until recently, there have been very few well-defined programs with clear evidence of beneficial outcomes.

All this comes at a time when health care is confronting constrained resources and consumer and regulatory demands that require us to look very carefully at the costs as well as the quality of our care and interventions. To achieve the appropriate balance, our practice needs to be increasingly based on evidence, moving us from "I believe this should work" to that which we know does work. This volume and its authors greatly contribute to moving us toward this end. With broader discussion and use of evidenced-based practice, we can provide not only the most appropriate utilization of resources, but more importantly, the best possible care for our patients.

Nancy Gibbs, MD
Kaiser Permanente Continuing Care Department
Downey, California

Acknowledgments

I am pleased to bring forward a compendium of research, knowledge, and examples of translational efforts in moving research to practice. The movement toward evidence-based practices is gaining growing attention, yet there is little understanding about how to gather information about model programs and even less on how to adapt them for practice. With the assistance of my esteemed colleagues and fellow contributors to this volume, we are excited to offer preliminary insights into the world of evidence-based health practices targeting community dwelling older adults. I would also like to thank the contributors for their dedication to this publication and especially for their perseverance and commitment in advancing health practice through research and dissemination. It is through the expertise and inquiry of researchers, practitioners, policymakers, and academics, such as these contributors, that lends itself to innovation and discovery of best practices.

I would also like to thank several organizations that have provided unique leadership in developing, testing, and implementing new and better models of care for older adults including Partners in Care Foundation, U.S. Department of Health and Human Services, Administration on Aging, University of Southern California Andrus School of Gerontology and School of Social Work, Kaiser Permanente, Boston University's Institute for Geriatric Social Work, the Center for Successful Aging, California State University, Fullerton, and the Archstone Foundation. The support and guidance of these organizations is instrumental in advancing this valuable work.

Susan M. Enguídanos, MPH, PhD

Evidence-Based Health Practice:
Knowing and Using What Works
for Older Adults

Mary Altpeter, PhD, MSW, MPA
Lucinda Bryant, PhD, MSHA, MBA
Ellen Schneider, MBA
Nancy Whitelaw, PhD, MS

SUMMARY. Community-based health care agencies are facing demands for improved outcomes, cost-effective programming, and higher customer satisfaction. Implementing evidence-based health interventions and programs can help to address these challenges. This article provides an overview of evidence-based health practice, including the definition and advantages of this approach, other key terms and concepts inherent to evidence-based practice, and the tasks and steps necessary to

---

Mary Altpeter is Associate Director for Program Development, Research Associate Professor of Social Work, University of North Carolina Institute on Aging, 720 Martin Luther King, Jr. Blvd., Campus Box 1030, Chapel Hill, NC 27599-1030 (E-mail: mary_altpeter@unc.edu). Lucinda Bryant is Assistant Professor, Department of Preventive Medicine and Biometrics, University of Colorado at Denver and Health Sciences Center, 4200 East Ninth Avenue, Box C-245, Denver, CO 80262 (E-mail: lucinda.bryant@uchsc.edu). Ellen Schneider is Program Manager, The University of North Carolina Institute on Aging, 720 Martin Luther King, Jr. Blvd., Campus Box 1030, Chapel Hill, NC 27599-1030 (E-mail: eschneider@schsr.unc.edu). Nancy Whitelaw is Director, Center for Healthy Aging, National Council on the Aging, 300 D Street, SW, Suite 801, Washington, DC 20024 (E-mail: nancy.whitelaw@ncoa.org).

[Haworth co-indexing entry note]: "Evidence-Based Health Practice: Knowing and Using What Works for Older Adults." Altpeter, Mary et al. Co-published simultaneously in *Home Health Care Services Quarterly* (The Haworth Press, Inc.) Vol. 25, No. 1/2, 2006, pp. 1-11; and: *Evidence-Based Interventions for Community Dwelling Older Adults* (ed: Susan M. Enguídanos) The Haworth Press, Inc., 2006, pp. 1-11. Single or multiple copies of this article are available for a fee from The Haworth Document Delivery Service [1-800-HAWORTH, 9:00 a.m. - 5:00 p.m. (EST). E-mail address: docdelivery@haworthpress.com].

its implementation. The article concludes with a list of resources to help health care providers learn about, plan, and implement evidence-based health interventions and programs. *[Article copies available for a fee from The Haworth Document Delivery Service: 1-800-HAWORTH. E-mail address: <docdelivery@haworthpress.com> Website: <http://www.HaworthPress.com>*
© *2006 by The Haworth Press, Inc. All rights reserved.]*

KEYWORDS. Evidence base, evidenced-based health practice, older adults, public health, fidelity, ecological approach

INTRODUCTION

This special volume provides community-based aging services professionals with an overview of evidence-based health practice and examples of its applicability and importance to their work. Learning the process of planning and implementing evidence-based programs will offer providers better tools to address the mounting organizational challenges they face today: increasing competition; capitated reimbursement and escalating costs; and demands for improved outcomes, cost effectiveness, and customer satisfaction (Sobolewski & Marren, 2000). Evidence-based practice also provides a vehicle for providers to deliver high quality services to their older and frail clients, helping them to preserve or restore function, maintain or improve physical and mental health status, and prevent or delay institutionalization.

This introductory article explains why providers should consider evidence-based practice, defines this approach, and lays out its component tasks and steps. It ends with a list of references–publications, audiovisual materials, and websites–for those readers who wish to investigate this topic in greater depth. Succeeding articles in this collection cover a range of topics that describe methods for collecting evidence about actual program benefits that can alter prevailing practice beliefs and support positive change in service delivery; discuss evidence-based strategies for various health interventions; and detail the challenges, obstacles, and practice knowledge gained in the application of evidence-based approaches germane to home health care and community settings. Specifically, the authors describe and illustrate the following:

• How to move from tacit knowledge to evidence-based practice in geriatric case management (Enguídanos and Jamison)

- The translation of the original research on a medications management intervention in a home health care program to replication in a community-based waiver care management program (Alkema and Frey)
- A comprehensive assessment of evidence-based falls prevention intervention strategies (Pynoos et al.)
- The implementation of an evidence-based physical activity intervention for frail elders (Wieckowski and Simmons)
- The adaptation of an evidence-based model of depression care for population-wide use (Geron and Keefe)
- A comprehensive review of the prevalence and characteristics of depression among older adults, evidence-based interventions, multi-level barriers to care, effective strategies, and key research-to-practice issues (Ell)
- The barriers and facilitators encountered in replicating an evidence-based palliative care model (Davis et al.)

The timing of this publication is ideal. There is growing national recognition of the importance of evidence-based programming for older adults. The Administration on Aging has established a National Resource Center on Evidence-Based Prevention at the National Council on the Aging to support widespread adoption of such programming. In addition, the Centers for Disease Control and Prevention offer valuable expertise through the Healthy Aging Research Network, and several foundations are supporting specific projects such as those described here.

We hope that the varied topics presented within these pages will provoke your thinking about key questions, such as "What programs do we know work in real-world community settings?" and "In which population does a particular program work best?" We start with why the evidence-based practice approach is vital to addressing these questions.

WHY CONSIDER EVIDENCE-BASED PRACTICE FOR OLDER ADULTS?

Older age can bring increased health-related risks that include physical inactivity, poor diet, obesity, falls, depression, mismanagement of medications, lack of preventive care, and improper management of chronic diseases. Community-based aging service providers can offer valuable experience and resources to assist broad-based community partnerships with health promotion and chronic disease management interventions (Beattie, Whitelaw, Mettler, & Turner, 2003). However, despite this expertise, providers of care to active or home-based older adults may find it difficult to *prove* that their programs are efficient or effective, or make tangible, positive, and sustained differences in the lives of their clients. Organizations may find it relatively straightforward to report survey results and anecdotes about client satisfaction and to document impressive levels of units of service. However, if challenged to show proof of program effectiveness, providers may be tempted to fall back on practical experience and say, "Trust me, I've been working with my clients for years and I can tell what's working." These efforts, however, do not respond to the questions at the heart of the issue:

- Does the program truly produce measurable benefits in the older adult population?
- As a service provider, can I be sure that my program does not cause harm or waste limited resources?
- If my program uses untested or unproven approaches or evaluation measures, how can I determine the causes of its success or failure?
- If my program fails to produce the intended results, how can I pinpoint the problem? For example, did I choose the wrong type of intervention? Target a population that either did not need or could not benefit from the intervention? Use incorrect or inadequate measures to evaluate the program?

Evidence-based practice addresses these questions as well as other issues such as resources and sustainability. Table 1 summarizes many of the advantages of using an evidence-based approach. Using scientific evidence, providers can make better decisions about which populations to serve, how to assist them, and whether specific programs should be defended and continued. Given these benefits, what then constitutes evidence-based practice?

WHAT ARE THE COMPONENTS
OF EVIDENCE-BASED PRACTICE?

To explain *evidence-based practice*, we first need to understand that the acquisition of an evidence base requires a population perspective, even though practice occurs at the individual level. The field of public

TABLE 1. Advantages of an Evidence-Based Approach

1. Increases the likelihood of successful outcomes when providers move away from decision-making that relies too heavily on history, anecdotes, and/or pressure from policy makers

2. Enhances the ability to identify common health indicators and match health programs to those risks and conditions

3. Makes it easier to defend or expand an existing program

4. Increases effective use of resources

5. Provides hard data to advocate for new programs

6. Generates new knowledge about "what works" and "how to do it" that can help others

Note. Adapted from "Module 1: Introduction to Evidence-Based Health," The Community Guide, 2004, at http://www.thecommunityguide.org/Training%20Resources/default.htm.

health provides a basis for understanding this *epidemiological perspective* (i.e., focusing on the population rather than the individual and emphasizing both prevention and treatment). Public health addresses the health and well-being of a community, with the goal of creating and sustaining the proper conditions to support people's mental and physical health (Institute of Medicine, 1988). Public health takes an *ecological* approach that includes people, families and social networks, communities, systems of services, social and cultural norms, laws and political processes, the built and natural environments, and the interactions and reciprocal influences among them. An ecological intervention thus targets and links activities across many levels, from the individual to the community and to society as a whole.

As an example, later in this volume, Geron and Keefe discuss care management and treatment planning as not only individual-level assessment of several domains of a person's physical and emotional health but also the examination of system-level factors to assure maximum access to community resources and support. Ell enumerates multiple levels of intervention strategies and activities in her discussion of depression care. Davis and colleagues further apply the socio-ecological framework in describing the staff, managerial and organizational contextual factors that facilitate or impede the adoption by agencies of innovative evidence-base programs in palliative care.

Falls prevention programs such as *A Matter of Balance* provide a good illustration of the multi-level ecological approach incorporated into a program implementation strategy. This program is designed to improve knowledge and behavior of at-risk individuals, assess built environments for hazards that may cause falls, and promote relationships between senior centers and relevant community and health care organizations to develop, implement, evaluate, and disseminate falls prevention information (Administration on Aging, 2004). For additional discussion of multi-level falls prevention intervention strategies, see the article by Pynoos and colleagues.

The term *evidence* refers to a body of facts or information that evaluates the validity ("truth") of something–for instance, reports of the health risks or conditions of older adults in a community or assertions about the value of a particular health-related program. The term *evidence base* encompasses several components that include (a) the results of a systematic identification and review of the relevant body of facts or information addressing a well-defined question, (b) the methods and detailed procedures for addressing that question, (c) the measurement of outcomes, and (d) a description of the characteristics and environment of a target population affected by the question. The purpose of an evidence base is to provide knowledge of effective content and methods that can be translated into specific interventions that providers can apply to improve the health of individuals and populations.

Experts talk about three types of *evidence* (Brownson, Baker, Leet, & Gillespie, 2003; Rychetnik, Hawe, Waters, Barratt, & Frommer, 2004):

1. Evidence about the health issue that supports the statement, "*Something* should be done."
2. Evidence about a tested program intervention or model that has been shown to address the health issue that supports the statement, "*This* should be done."
3. Evidence about the design, context, and attractiveness of the program to participants and other community stakeholders that supports the statement, "*How* this should be done."

The concept of evidence, then, applies not only to confirming the existence of a specific health risk or condition, but also to matching a tested intervention or model with the health risk or condition and specifying how to tailor the intervention to work in the target population. Combining all of these concepts, *evidence-based practice* is a process of planning, implementing, and evaluating programs that consider health issues in an ecological context and have a foundation in *tested models or interventions*. Later in this volume, Ell suggests the term "empirically supported" to encompass the ecological span of factors that affect evidence-based practice, including: "patient care seeking and adherence behavior; provider knowledge, clinical decision making and care management skills; health care system design or redesign; and organizational incentives and resources that lead to the implementation of evidence based practice and program guidelines, and empirically derived quality monitoring indicators" (p. xx).

Thus, the evidence-based practice approach consists of a series of steps to guide service planners and providers through identification of important risk factors and health conditions, selection of the target population, program planning decisions, partnership building, implementation actions, selection of program quality and cost evaluation measures, and sustainability considerations. In essence, evidence-based program planning and implementation activities create the bridge between intervention research and practice.

WHAT ARE THE TASKS AND STEPS FOR EVIDENCE-BASED PRACTICE?

Table 2 lists the tasks and steps that guide evidence-based practice. These tasks and steps are adapted from the evidence-based public health literature (Brownson et al., 2003; Kahan & Goodstadt, 2001). The first task involves identifying health risks and issues important to older adults and then investigating and selecting appropriate interventions that have been proven to be effective with the target population. A suitable program will need translation from the identified, often research-based intervention's original application (i.e., with a specific test group under controlled "laboratory-like" settings using tightly monitored protocols). To accomplish this translation, providers need to understand the *core elements*, or functional "active ingredients," of the intervention that must be present to make it work. These immutable core elements differ from *key characteristics* of the intervention methods. Key characteristics are those flexible components of the intervention that should be adapted, such as recruitment methods or modification of educational materials (e.g., the size of font or the language level) in order to be culturally appropriate for the population being served (Hawe, Shiell, & Riley, 2004; Washington State Department of Health, 2004). Adherence to the core elements of an intervention, called *fidelity*, is central to evidence-based practice.

Effective programming requires not only an evidence base for the program, but also evidence-based evaluation. This evaluation occurs at two levels, measuring both implementation (process evaluation) and ef-

TABLE 2. Evidence-Based Health Practice

Tasks	Steps
Identify an important health issue and population at risk	1. Review epidemiological and other data to identify key health/functional conditions and risk factors for older adults in the community
	2. Specify the characteristics and contexts (e.g., factors such as income, education, culture, geographic location, accessibility to services) of the population at risk, providers, and the broader community
Identify effective intervention(s)	3. Systematically identify and review relevant research and information on proven interventions or models that address the targeted conditions or risk factors
Select an intervention	4. Select a proven evidence-based intervention or model (from those identified in Step 3) that will be appropriate for the target community, suitable for adoption by providers, and feasible given available provider and community resources
Translate the intervention into a practice	5. Translate the tested intervention or model into a practice suitable for provider implementation while maintaining fidelity (i.e., the accurate and faithful reproduction of the core elements of the evidence-based intervention in the design and implementation of the practice)
	6. Recruit and retain high risk, older adults from the target population who can benefit from the intervention
	7. Implement the translated practice, maintaining fidelity to the core elements and design established in Step 5, while adapting key characteristics (e.g., outreach methods, language level, and font size of educational materials) to the needs and characteristics of the target population
Evaluate the program	8. Plan goals for process and outcomes evaluation, design instruments and protocols for data collection, and assign responsibilities for evaluation
	9. Provide midcourse feedback on program operations and implementation and decide what adjustments (if any) need to be made
	10. Measure and evaluate program delivery and outcomes to assess the effectiveness of the program or model and inform the next cycle of planning
Sustain the program	11. Determine the information, activities, and resources that maintainance of successful individual and provider outcomes will require. Ask the following questions: • What are the desired long-term effects for participants? • How can these effects be supported programmatically? • What resources will be needed to maintain desired individual-level outcomes and institutionalize the program?

fects (outcomes evaluation). Outcomes evaluation may take place at both individual and community levels to assess the changes in program participants' learning, health behaviors, and health status, as well as the effects of the program on community health status. Sustainability, like evaluation, concerns both the individual and the program. At the individual level, if an evidence-based practice produces positive short-term outcomes, then it is important to take the next step to plan for long-term lasting effects on health status. In addition, evaluation data that document successful evidence-based practice outcomes can serve as the basis for defending and advocating for the sustainment and institutionalization of the program.

Providers need to understand the fundamentals of the process, but as Wieckowski and Simmons note, they also must evaluate their readiness to implement evidence-based health programming. The National Council on the Aging has developed a readiness checklist which is available at the NCOA Center for Healthy Aging web site: http://www.healthy agingprograms.org/. Another tool for assessing readiness for implementing evidence-based health programs is available on the RE-AIM website (http://www.re-aim.org/). RE-AIM is a framework for evidence-based practice, and the acronym stands for *Reach*, the number, proportion, and representativeness of individuals who are willing to participate in a given program or intervention; *Efficacy or Effectiveness*, the impact of the intervention on important outcomes, including potential negative effects, quality of life, and economic outcomes; *Adoption*, the number, proportion, and representativeness of settings and intervention agents that are willing to initiate the intervention or program; *Implementation*, the fidelity to the various elements of an intervention's protocol; and *Maintenance*, the extent to which a program becomes institutionalized or part of the routine organizational practices and policies, and at the individual level, the sustainment of health outcomes 6 or more months after the most recent intervention contact (RE-AIM.org, 2004). The RE-AIM framework was created by a group of researchers in the National Institutes of Health Behavioral Change Consortium for planning health interventions and measuring their impact in community settings. Alkema and Frey illustrate the translation of a medication management intervention into a community-based program, using the Promoting Action on Research Implementation in Health Services revised framework (PARIHS) (Rycroft-Malone et al., 2002). This framework is built on three essential and interacting factors–evidence, context, and facilitation–and it provides another tool for understanding and addressing the necessary elements for implementing effective evidence-based strategies. Additional resources and tools are presented in the Audiovisual and Internet Resources sections at the end of this article.

CONCLUSION

With the exponential growth of the older population and the desire of older adults to remain in their homes, the need to identify and implement cost-effective and high quality programs presents a both urgent and daunting challenge for health care providers. Implementation of evidence-based practice approaches promises help in meeting these challenges. Aging services providers, with their reach into communities of all sizes, have the capacity to meet the demand. The articles that follow present additional conceptual approaches, practice tips, and tools to support providers' efforts.

REFERENCES

Administration on Aging. (2004). *Evidence-based disease prevention grants program: Falls prevention.* Retrieved November 21, 2004, from http://www.aoa.gov/prof/evidence/evidence.asp

Beattie, B. L., Whitelaw, N., Mettler, M., & Turner, D. (2003). A vision for older adults and health promotion. *American Journal of Health Promotion, 18*(2), 200-204.

Brownson, R. C., Baker, E. A., Leet, T. L., & Gillespie, K. N. (2003). *Evidence-based public health.* New York: Oxford University Press.

Hawe, P., Shiell, A., & Riley, T. (2004). Complex interventions: How "out of control" can a randomised controlled trial be? *British Medical Journal, 328,* 1561-1563.

Institute of Medicine (U.S.), Committee for the Study of the Future of Public Health. (1988). *The future of public health.* Washington, DC: National Academy Press.

Kahan, B., & Goodstadt, M. (2001). The interactive domain model of best practices in health promotion: Developing and implementing a best practices approach to health promotion. *Health Promotion Practice, 2*(1), 43-67.

National Council on the Aging. (2004). *Partnering to promote healthy aging: Creative best practice community partnerships.* Retrieved December 17, 2004, from http://www.ncoa.org/Downloads/FINALHApartnerships%5Fweb%2Epdf

RE-AIM.org. (2004). *What is RE-AIM?* Retrieved December 18, 2004, from http://www.re-aim.org/2003/defined.html

Rychetnik, L., Hawe, P., Waters, E., Barratt, A., & Frommer, M. (2004). A glossary for evidence based public health. *Journal of Epidemiology & Community Health, 58*(7), 538-545.

Rycroft-Malone, J., Kitson, A. Harvey, G., McCormack, B., Seers, K., Titchen, A. & Estabrooks, C. (2002). Ingredients for change: Revisiting a conceptual framework. *Quality & Safety in Health Care, 11*(2): 174-180.

Sobolewski, S., & Marren, J. (2000, Winter). Home care and the new economy: Creating a new model for service delivery. *Care Management Journals, 2*(4), 248-252.

Washington State Department of Health. (2004). *Effective HIV interventions and strategies.* Retrieved November 21, 2004, from http://www.doh.wa.gov/cfh/hiv_aids/ Prev_Edu/Effective_Interventions/Eff_Int_Doc.pdf

AUDIOVISUAL RESOURCES

Evidence-Based Public Health Practice Workshop on The Guide to Community Preventive Services, Center for the Evaluative Clinical Sciences at Dartmouth (April 21, 2004). http://www.thecommunityguide. org/Training%20Resources/default.htm
   Module 1: Introduction to evidence-based health
   Module 2: Mechanics of evidence reviews
   Module 3: Applying evidence-based resources in public health practice

INTERNET RESOURCES

Administration on Aging Evidence-Based Disease Prevention Grants Program
http://www.aoa.gov/prof/evidence/evidence.asp

Cochrane Collaboration
http://www.cochrane.org/index0.htm

Health Development Agency (HDA) Evidence Base
http://www.hda-online.org.uk/evidence/

National Council on the Aging Center for Healthy Aging
http://www.healthyagingprograms.org/

Public Health Data Standards Consortium Web-Based Resource Center
http://www.phdatastandards.info/knowresources/tutorials/tutorials.htm

RE-AIM.org
http://www.re-aim.org/

The Community Toolbox
http://ctb.ku.edu/

The Guide to Preventive Community Services
http://www.thecommunityguide.org/

The Office of Disease Prevention and Health Promotion, Office of Public Health and Science, Office of the Secretary, U.S. Department of Health and Human Services
http://www.health.gov/phfunctions/public.htm

Moving from Tacit Knowledge to Evidence-Based Practice: The Kaiser Permanente Community Partners Study

Susan M. Enguídanos, MPH, PhD
Paula M. Jamison, BA, MA Candidate

SUMMARY. For several decades both medical and social work practices have failed to consistently include measures to determine the effectiveness of their care and practices. This is especially true of care management practices. With the growth and aging of our population, this is of particular concern when many of our resources for older adults are channeled into services such as geriatric care management. This article describes a randomized controlled trial that tested the effectiveness of four levels of geriatric care management. Results from this study did not support the tacit knowledge of the clinicians in terms of the effectiveness of their practices. This article describes the study methods and results, and how evidence from this study impacted subsequent service provided by geriatric care managers. *[Article copies available for a fee from The Haworth Document Delivery Service: 1-800-HAWORTH. E-mail address: <docdelivery@haworthpress.*

Susan M. Enguídanos is Research Director, Partners in Care Foundation, 6131 E. Peabody, Long Beach, CA 90808 (E-mail: senguidanos@picf.org). Paula M. Jamison is Program Manager, Partners in Care Foundation, 2505 E. First Street, Long Beach, CA 90803 (E-mail: pjamison@picf.org).

[Haworth co-indexing entry note]: "Moving from Tacit Knowledge to Evidence-Based Practice: The Kaiser Permanente Community Partners Study." Enguídanos, Susan M., and Paula M. Jamison. Co-published simultaneously in *Home Health Care Services Quarterly* (The Haworth Press, Inc.) Vol. 25, No. 1/2, 2006, pp. 13-31; and: *Evidence-Based Interventions for Community Dwelling Older Adults* (ed: Susan M. Enguídanos) The Haworth Press, Inc., 2006, pp. 13-31. Single or multiple copies of this article are available for a fee from The Haworth Document Delivery Service [1-800-HAWORTH, 9:00 a.m. - 5:00 p.m. (EST). E-mail address: docdelivery@haworthpress.com].

Available online at http://www.haworthpress.com/web/HHC
doi:10.1300/J027v25n01_02

KEYWORDS. Care management, evidence-based, geriatric care, social work, health, randomized trial, effectiveness, practice

INTRODUCTION

Evidence-based medicine as defined by the Institute of Medicine is "the integration of best researched evidence and clinical expertise with patient values" (IOM 2001, p. 147). The medical field desires to achieve a point in which clinical practice is based upon the findings of empirical research; however, this is only a recently developed goal. Claridge and Fabian (2005) report in their article describing the history of evidence-based medicine that this term only came into existence in the 1990s. Several studies have documented that a large majority of clinical decision-making is not typically based in findings from evidence-based research but on tacit knowledge (Carter, 1996; Claridge & Fabian, 2005; Pryjmachuk, 1996). Pryjmachuk (1996) suggests that although nurses may be familiar with theory, they lack an understanding of the importance of its application in practice. In her review of literature citing barriers to the implementation of research findings in practice, Carter (1996) discusses evidence that implies that much of nursing practice is based on ritual rather than empirical evidence. One of the critical obstacles in supporting the use of research findings into practice is the ability to translate results into the application of clinical practice (Rosen, 2000). This is evident not only among medical clinicians but in the field of social work in healthcare as well.

The importance of shifting practice guided by tacit knowledge to evidence-based knowledge is receiving increased attention in the field of social work. A literature review found that only fifteen percent of all research studies conducted on social work interventions were controlled trials (Rosen, Proctor, & Staudt, 1999). In addition, only one in seven percent of research articles in social work actually tested the effectiveness of a social work intervention (Rosen et al., 1999). Among the studies that have documented the efficacy of social work interventions using controlled trials, few have attempted to isolate which aspects of a social work intervention have the greatest impact on positive outcomes (Gorey,

1996; National Chronic Care Consortium (NCCC), 1997; Parker, 1997; Reid, Kenaley, Colvin, & Fortune, 2004).

Social work interventions in healthcare typically assess several domains of a person's physical and emotional health in order to identify how to appropriately conduct their treatment. In addition to the individual level assessment, system level factors are examined in order to assure maximum access to community resources and support is established. This type of intervention is typically identified as care management. Care management consists of "comprehensive client-oriented needs assessment to identify unmet needs or problems inhibiting secure and independent living in a home environment, followed by developing and periodically reviewing a care service plan" (*http://www.intergens. com/glossary.html*). Care management models are widely used to assist various populations such as persons with chronic illness, the elderly, and disabled. This type of intervention is most prevalently used among the elderly due to the complex medical and social problems that they face.

Despite the prevalence of case management practice, there has been little evidence of efficacy and effectiveness in the application of these models. What studies exist on geriatric care models often lack rigor or contain methodological weaknesses that result in questionable findings (Lee, Mackenzie, Dudley-Brown, & Chin, 1998). In the last few years, several studies on the efficacy of geriatric case management have been conducted using experimental designs with randomized control groups (Boult, Rassen, Rassen, Moore, & Robison, 2000; Engelhardt et al., 1996; Fordyce, Bardole, Romer, Soghikian, & Fireman, 1997; Gagnon, Schein, McVey, & Bergman, 1999; Leveille et al., 1998; Long & Marshall, 1999; Marshall, Long, Voss, Demma, & Skerl, 1999; Morishita, Boult, Boult, Smith, & Pacala, 1998; Nalyor et al., 1999; Schore, Brown, & Cheh, 1999; Weuve, Boult, & Morishita, 2000). These projects aimed to improve health and functioning, reduce medical service use, decrease rates of depression, and increase client satisfaction, among other goals. Results of these studies are inconsistent, with some reporting decreased rates of service use (Leveille et al., 1998; Nalyor et al., 1999), others reported no difference or increase of service use (Boult et al., 2000; Fordyce et al., 1997; Gagnon et al., 1999; Long & Marshall, 1999; Schore et al., 1999). Similarly, levels of satisfaction and functioning for the case management group also varied across studies (Gagnon et al., 1999; Marshall et al., 1999; Morishita et al., 1998). Moreover, none of the studies measuring depression level were actually able to impact depression through their interventions (Engelhardt et al., 1996; Leveille et al., 1998; Nalyor et al., 1999).

This paper discusses the results of a randomized controlled trial evaluating the effectiveness of a geriatric care management model delivered in a managed care setting. Reid et al. (2004) discuss the need to test the efficacy of social work interventions and determine what components of these models are effective in reaching intended outcomes. This study documents the first step in integrating evidence-based practice into the social work clinical setting. It is necessary to first test the efficacy of current models of care in order to demonstrate if clinicians' tacit knowledge about interventions produces definitive results.

METHODS

In 1998 Kaiser Permanente (KP) in partnership with Partners in Care Foundation (Partners) and the L.A. County and L.A. City Area Agencies on Aging (AAA), received a four-year grant from the California HealthCare Foundation's Program for Elders in Managed Care. The purpose of the award was to test models of Geriatric Care Management and to determine whether geriatric care management plus a brief payment intervention (up to $2,000 of designated paid services such as in-home supportive services, transportation, respite or medical equipment) would lower medical costs, improve satisfaction with care, increase care plan adherence and improve perceived quality of life. An additional aim of this project was to determine if improved collaboration between KP and AAA agencies would result in improved patient outcomes.

This research project built upon a model of care developed in KP's TriCentral service area in which the goal of the model was to create a continuum of care matching the level and type of services, whether preventive, restorative or palliative to the members' needs. The original concept for this project arose from observations in clinical practice that significant barriers existed that prevented frail elderly from accessing key home and community-based services (HCBS) necessary to prevent decline, promote optimal health status and quality of life, and reduce the need for use of acute care services. These barriers to access were hypothesized to be lack of knowledge by frail elderly and their families about available services, resistance to accepting formal services in the home, and lack of financial resources or unwillingness to pay for services. A further assumption was that if these barriers could be lowered or eliminated, we would see improvements in health status and functioning for frail elderly, and lower total medical care costs.

Another primary purpose of the study was to gain evidence of the effectiveness of the geriatric care management program in improving patient outcomes and reducing health care costs. Study investigators, geriatric care management leaders and staff had tacit knowledge of the effectiveness of these practices but did not have the research findings to support their intuition. Through this research project, the clinicians expected to gather the evidence they had long sought demonstrating the effectiveness of the program.

The specific aims of the study were to determine whether and to what extent geriatric care management and/or a purchase of service intervention would lower barriers to access to home and community-based services; and in doing so, lower medical care costs, increase satisfaction with care, improve care plan compliance, and improve members' perception of quality of life. The following research questions will be addressed in this paper:

1. Frail older patients receiving geriatric care management or geriatric care management with a purchase of service will demonstrate higher satisfaction with their care compared to similar groups receiving telephone assistance and information and referral by mail.
2. Frail older patients receiving geriatric care management or geriatric care management with purchase of service will perceive a higher quality of life (superior clinical and functional outcomes) compared to members receiving telephone assistance and information and referral by mail.
3. Frail older patients receiving geriatric care management or geriatric care management with purchase of service will demonstrate lower medical care costs compared to patients receiving telephone assistance and information and referral by mail.

Design

The study design employed was a randomized control trial. Study participants were randomly assigned to one of four groups: information via mail, telephone care management, geriatric care management, or geriatric care management with purchase of service. The GCM team consisted of two bachelor level social workers who provided telephone care management and six social workers and nurses who conducted in-home care management.

Subjects

All patients referred for Geriatric Care Management program services were screened for program eligibility. Referrals were made to GCM by a KP health care professional, community service agency, caregiver or family member, or through self-referral. In addition, referrals were made using a Health Screening Form (HSF), a self-report instrument to predict elderly members at risk for frailty in the coming year (Brody, Johnson, & Ried, 1997). In 1998, Health Status Forms were mailed to the TriCentral region's existing members over the age of 75. Those identified as frail were referred to the GCM program for assessment.

Eligibility Criteria

To be eligible for the study, a KP member must be 65 years of age or older and meet at least one of the following five criteria:

- Had more than 3 emergency room visits or 3 hospitalizations in the past 12 months
- Utilized more than two medical office visits in past 3 months
- Have one or more ADL deficiencies as measured by the Katz Index of ADL (Katz & Akpom, 1976)
- Have cognitive impairment as measured by a score of less than 25 on the Telephone Interview for Cognitive Status (TICS) (Brandt, Spencer, & Folstein, 1996)
- Have one or more IADL deficiencies

In addition, the member must meet one of the following criteria:

- Does not have a caregiver to provide assistance with ADLs or IADLs deficiencies
- Has severe behavior problems as measured by a shortened version of the Memory and Behavior Problems Checklist (Teri et al., 1992).
- Has a caregiver reporting caregiver stress/burden as measured by a score of 5 or greater on a shortened version of the Burden Interview (Zarit & Zarit, 1983).

Study Groups

The four levels of care tested included: Information and Referral Assistance, Telephone Care Management, Geriatric Care Management, and Geriatric Care Management with a Purchase of Service Benefit. These four levels of interventions were selected because they represent the full continuum of care management practices. The Information and Referral intervention reflected the then current minimum level of care management practice within KP and was expected to serve as a control group.

Information and Referral Assistance: This group received information and referrals via mail tailored to their needs and specific geographical location. This information and referral package was assembled by telephone care managers based on the needs identified through the telephone interview.

Telephone Care Management (TCM): This was a short-term telephone-based intervention conducted by bachelor's level social workers. The patient was called within 48 working hours of the referral into the department. The TCM reviewed the history of utilization of KP systems and services, recent illnesses, diagnoses, and current medications prior to contacting the patient. The TCM then spoke with patient and primary caregiver and confirmed initial assessment information, discussed and facilitated needed services, referrals, and other needs with patient/caregiver and encouraged access to these services. Finally, a follow-up letter was sent to the patient reiterating the information provided via telephone. A telephone follow-up call to the patient was made at two to four weeks following initial contact. For each case, approximately four to five telephone contacts were made with patients, family members, community service agencies, and KP service providers over a four-week period. The total time spent on each case averaged 45 minutes.

Geriatric Care Management (GCM): This intervention was provided by a care manager who was either a Registered Nurse or Master's Level Clinical Social Worker. The GCM intervention was similar to the Telephone Case Management intervention in its goals and objectives. However, the GCM intervention was more comprehensive in that it included in-home visits and ongoing coordination, monitoring and follow-up. Upon assignment of a new case, the care manager conducted an in-home assessment with the client to determine or verify the health-related problems and needs of the member. This face-to-face assessment expanded upon the telephone assessment used to determine eligibility by verifying the previous information collected and collecting additional information about environmental conditions and home safety. In addition, data were collected regarding need for and availability of equipment, nature of family or neighborhood support, status of legal planning, eligibility for entitlement programs, and psychosocial needs. Based on the information collected in both assessments, a care plan was developed to address health-related and psychosocial needs and included target dates for problem resolution.

The initial care plan was reviewed at case conference team meetings with the GCM Team that included a geriatrician and Assistant Department Manager, and then reviewed with the member and their caregiver. The team provided care recommendations on issues such as treatment options, potential medications adjustments, assistance with problem solving on complicated home safety situations, and other information that would enhance the development and implementation of the care plan. Following review of the care plan, the care manager worked with the patient and the family to assist them in negotiating the KP system to address the identified needs, or to access services available from community agencies outside of the KP system.

The GCM intervention generally involved at least one in-home visit, several follow-up calls or visits with the patient or caregiver, and extensive coordination among both community and KP service providers. The care manager spent approximately 20 hours on each case over an average of 8-9 months time, with the bulk of the time invested within the first three months of care management.

GCM with Purchase of Service (POS) Capability: This intervention included all of the elements of the GCM intervention with the addition of up to $2,000 of designated, paid services available within the first six months of geriatric care management enrollment. Provision of these funds was intended to facilitate initial implementation of the care plan, and overcome barriers of access to home and community-based services. The goals of care plan implementation were the same: to stabilize or improve health status or prevent decline.

Care managers were expected to use AAA or other local and state-funded public programs to implement care plans where possible and appropriate. If the member was not eligible for these programs, or if a waiting list exists, POS funds could be used to provide designated services from a list of approved agencies or vendors. POS designated services are listed below and also included other special needs considered critical for maintaining or improving health status, or preventing a crisis or decline in the patient or in the caregiver. Specific designated services include In-Home Supportive Services (e.g., personal care, homemaker/

chore, home delivered meals), medical equipment, transportation, and respite care.

Data Collection

Data was collected from both patient interviews and from the KP service utilization databases. Interviews were conducted via telephone at study enrollment and at 12 months following enrollment. The telephone interview protocol was used to gather demographic data, physical status, satisfaction with services, quality of life, and caregiver burden. The following instruments were used:

Patient demographic data was collected via a demographic data sheet and included: age, ethnicity, marital status, gender, number of current medical conditions, education level, living situation, living arrangement, income level, and caregiver source.

Caregiver Burden. The Zarit and Zarit (Zarit & Zarit, 1983) burden interview was administered to collect information on caregiver burden and stress. The Burden Interview was designed to assess the stresses experienced by family caregivers of disabled persons. Internal reliability has been estimated with Cronbach's alpha at .88 (Hassinger, 1985) and validity at .71 (Gallagher, Rappaport, Benedict, Lovett, & Silven, 1985).

Service Use Data. At designated points throughout the study, service utilization data for each subject was collected from the KP mainframe database. Service data included number of Emergency Department visits, physician office visits, hospital days, skilled nursing facility days, home health and palliative visits, and days on Hospice. Service costs were calculated by taking the base service per day, plus cost for each service type and adding in related physician costs.

Functioning. The Katz Activities of Daily Living Scale was used to measure functioning. The Katz Index of ADL (Katz & Akpom, 1976) was developed to measure the physical functioning level of elderly and chronically ill patients. It assesses independence in six activities: bathing, dressing, toileting, transferring from bed to chair, continence, and feeding. The Independent Activities of Daily Living (IADL) Scale was used to assess independence in functioning of the following tasks: telephone use, traveling, cleaning, shopping, preparing meals, and medication and financial management.

Caregiver Availability/Adequacy. Each of the items measuring independence and functioning within the Katz and IADL Scales simultaneously measured the availability and adequacy of the patient's caregiver. Patients that reported a deficiency in functioning were then asked if a caregiver was available to assist them with their need and if so was their assistance adequate.

Caregiver Subjective Reaction to Patient Behaviors. The Memory and Behavior Problems Checklist (Zarit & Zarit, 1983) has also been condensed to measure how frequently a demented patient engaged in problematic behaviors and which problems were especially upsetting for caregivers. There are two parts to The Memory and Behavior Problems Checklist. The first part determines the frequency with which common problems occurred in the past week. The second part obtains the caregiver's subjective reaction to each problem.

Satisfaction with Services. The Reid-Gundlach Satisfaction with Services instrument was used in this study and has been successfully employed by 27 projects in the Health Resources and Service Administration (HRSA), Special Projects of National Significance study. The client satisfaction survey records the overall ratings of satisfaction with services, perception of service providers, and likelihood of positive recommendations of services to others.

Cognition. The Telephone Interview for Cognitive Status (TICS), a telephone cognition assessment tool, was used to measure cognitive impairment. This exam gives a brief assessment of the member's orientation to time and place, recall, and short-term memory (Brandt et al., 1996).

ANALYSES

Descriptive analyses were used to describe the sample. Chi-square and t-tests were used to determine if randomization was successful in terms of demographic and baseline characteristics. ANOVAS were conducted to compare group effects on dependent variables. Service use for each type of service (e.g., emergency department visit, hospitalization, physician visit, etc.) was examined as dichotomous variables with no significant differences in outcomes. Censoring models (such as probit and tobit models) were not used as some researchers have suggested that it is an inappropriate analytical strategy for count data such as service use (Breen, 1996; Orme & Buehler, 2001). Converting continuous data to censored data would result in a loss of information and richness offered from the interval level variable.

RESULTS

From May 2000 to September 2001, more than 1,400 senior members were referred to the GCM program; 156 (10.7%) refused the initial assessment and 35 (2.5%) were unable to be reached. Of those assessed, 50.4% were eligible for the study with 11.7% declining to participate. A total of 451 were randomized: 98 to information and referral, 113 to telephone care management, 117 to GCM, and 123 to GCM plus purchase of service.

Sample Description

All members receiving services were over the age of 65, with a mean age of 79. The sample was ethnically diverse as reflected in Table 1. A review of all baseline measures revealed that randomization was successful in assigning equivalent groups at baseline. There are no statistically significant differences between groups in terms of demographic variables, previous service use, number of self-reported medical conditions, living arrangements, and caregiver support. Additionally, no significant differences were detected between groups at baseline in terms of the dependent variables of interest in this study including activities of daily living, independent activities of daily living, baseline depression, and caregiver burden scores (see Table 1).

Attrition. Through the course of the project, several participants were lost to follow up. Attrition at 4 months was 6.6%; 20 died, 5 refused to complete the survey, 1 was unable to contact and 1 disenrolled from KP, and 3 were too frail/weak to participate in the telephone assessment. At 12 months, attrition increased to 40.7%; 39 died, 8 refused to complete the survey, 5 were unable to be contacted, 3 disenrolled from KP, and 99 were too frail/weak to participate in the telephone assessment. Attrition was equal across study groups. Examination of those who died/left compared to those who completed the study revealed that there were no significant differences in terms of baseline characteristics including demographic variables, health status, functioning, and prior service use.

Purchase of Service (POS). Use of the POS benefit was low. Although a total of 124 study participants were assigned to the POS group, only 54 participants actually used the benefit. More than half of the POS was used for homemaker services such as assistance with bathing and cleaning. Medical alert systems were the next frequently requested service, requested by 41 patients. Home repairs were requested by 22 and

TABLE 1. Sample Demographics by Study Group

Sample Demographics (percent)	Total (n = 452)	TCM (n = 113)	GCM (n = 117)	POS (n = 124)	I&R (n = 98)	P Value
Ethnicity:						.87
Caucasian	54	55	50	55	56	
African American	17	21	15	17	14	
Latino	17	14	18	17	20	
Asian/PI/Nat. American	4	2	5	4	6	
Other/Unknown	8	8	3	7	4	
Gender:						.92
Female	66	66	68	65	64	
Marital Status:						.70
Single	6	5	3	3	6	
Married	41	43	40	40	48	
Widowed	44	44	45	45	41	
Divorced/Separated	5	4	9	9	5	
Unknown	4	4	3	3		
Education:						.24
Less than high school	28	37	24	27	25	
High school grad	30	27	33	26	32	
Some college	17	14	13	20	20	
College grad or more	12	10	15	12	14	
Unknown	13	12	15	15	9	
Living situation:						
Own house	64	69	60	64	64	
Family member's home	13	11	16	12	14	
Apartment	9	9	7	12	8	
Senior living	3	3	4	2	2	
Other/Unknown	11	8	13	10	12	
Annual Income:						.41
Below $10,000	20	18	13	23	26	
$10,000 - $19,999	24	20	27	26	25	
$20,000 or more	18	34	18	28	16	
Unknown/Refused	38	28	42	23	33	
Live with:						.78
Alone	25	31	21	28	21	
Family member	63	57	65	60	71	
Paid caregiver	2	3	3	2	2	
Other/Unknown	10	9	11	10	6	
Primary caregiver:						
Spouse/Partner	31	30	31	28	38	
Child	33	31	32	37	34	
Paid caregiver	4	7	3	4	2	
Other/Unknown	32	32	35	31	28	

included minor home repairs such as installation of grab bars, rails and other minor home repairs.

Patient Level Outcomes by Study Group

The primary dependent variables (functioning, cognition, caregiver burden, and depression) were examined for differences within each study group from baseline to 12 months. Figure 1 and 2 contain the results of these analyses for ADLS and IADLs. There was no significant improvement or decline in functioning for any of the four study groups.

Similarly, Figure 3 contains the results of cognition level from baseline to 12 months. Higher cognition scores represent less impairment.

FIGURE 1. ADL Deficiencies Baseline to 12 Months

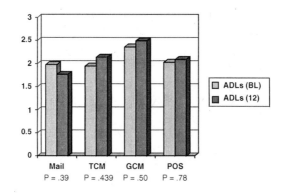

FIGURE 2. IADL Deficiencies Baseline to 12 Months

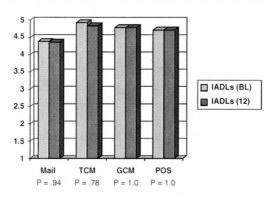

FIGURE 3. Cognitive Functioning Baseline to 12 Months

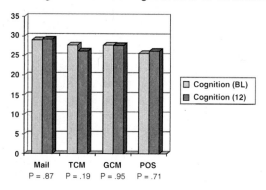

Again, there were no significant differences from baseline to 12 months among any of the study groups.

Depression levels within groups did vary. Among those in the POS and mail group, there were no significant within-group changes. The GCM only group demonstrated significant reductions in the level of depression from baseline to 12 months and the TCM group showed a strong trend toward lower depression levels at 12 months. Although statistically significant, the reduced depression level at 12 months for the GCM group was not clinically significant. See Figure 4.

All four intervention groups were able to demonstrate significant reduction of caregiver burden (see Figure 5). Figure 5 does not include the 40% who were too weak/frail or otherwise lost to follow-up as these individuals did not have caregivers available to provide caregiver or proxy information. Because the mail group had significantly reduced burden as well as the other groups, these results may be influenced by the data collection interview. Thus, the baseline, four month and 12 month interviews may have served as an intervention. Simply sharing their experience and stress during the interview may have reduced the stress level of the caregiver.

Service use for each type of service (e.g., emergency department visit, hospitalization, physician visit, etc.) was examined as dichotomous variables with no significant differences in outcomes. Analyses of costs of service use incurred from baseline to 12 months revealed no significant difference. An ANOVA was performed to determine if there were any difference in terms of level of service use at both 4 and 12 months among the four study groups. Results revealed no significant difference for any of the categories of services (see Table 2).

FIGURE 4. Depression Level from Baseline to 12 Months

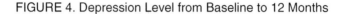

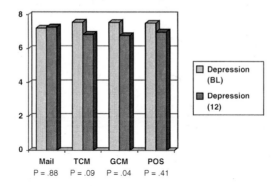

FIGURE 5. Caregiver Burden/Stress Baseline to 12 Months

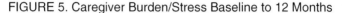

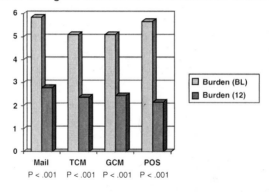

DISCUSSION

It is evident from the varied levels of analyses conducted and re-ported in this document that the interventions tested in this study did not have a significant impact on the dependent variables being tested. In fact, analyses demonstrated that all groups had equal outcomes at 12 months following study enrollment for nearly all variables examined. Hence, higher, more costly levels of GCM do not measurably improve patient outcomes in terms of functioning, service use, depression, care-giver burden, and cognition. Further, the added $2,000 benefit, which was not widely accepted and used by the study sample, did not help to improve patient outcomes. These findings are consistent with findings

TABLE 2. Service Use by Study Group (Percent Users)

Service	Mail		TCM		GCM		GCM+POS		p value	
	4 mth	12 mth	4 mth	12 mth	4 mth	12 mth	4 mth	12 mth	4	12
ER	42.2	50	40.2	46.8	48.2	58.6	41.0	58.1	.63	.43
Hospital	21.1	29.3	23.8	19.4	23.6	35.7	18.8	27.0	.78	.22
MD	96.7	93.1	89.2	90.3	93.6	91.6	94.9	93.2	.17	.92
SNF	7.8	10.3	5.0	4.8	9.1	14.3	9.4	10.8	.62	.36
Home Health	30	22.4	34.7	32.3	33.6	27.1	36.8	18.9	.79	.31

from other studies testing the effect of geriatric care management ser-vices (Boult et al., 2000; Fordyce et al., 1997; Gagnon et al., 1999; Long & Marshall, 1999; Marshall et al., 1999; Trella, 1993), where GCM was not indicative of reduced service use or improved patient functioning or depression. Moreover, consistent with the study conducted by (Fordyce et al., 1997; Long & Marshall, 1999), of geriatric care management ser-vices for patient at end of life, some of the analyses suggest that there was an upward trend in service use for the GCM groups. These results support the article by (Fordyce et al., 1997) that posits that more health services do not mean better care.

Further, the data obtained in this study revealed a high prevalence of depression among this population. The lowered levels of depression found at 12 months among those receiving TCM and GCM suggest that GCM may be an appropriate opportunity for intervention, although practices may be strengthened by addressing this depression through specific interventions as identified by Ell (2005) in this volume.

Shifting Beliefs and Practices

The findings of this study were key in shifting Kaiser leadership from reliance on tacit knowledge as their primary source of outcome mea-surement to the implementation of evidence-based measures to evaluate program effectiveness. The data presented provided irrefutable evi-dence that was in direct conflict with inherent beliefs about the benefits of the program services on older adults. However, the lack of significant results did not result in a lack of a significant contribution to geriatric care management practices. On the contrary, the findings revealed key areas of improvement in goals, practice, and education to be addressed in program.

This study illuminated several factors regarding GCM practice that must be taken into consideration in developing an effective intervention for this population. First, it is necessary to identify specific outcomes that you aim to address in your program. These outcomes must be explicit, realistic, and attainable. Next, the outcomes must be tied directly to the intervention provided. Thus, there must be evidence (or minimally a theoretical framework) that links the intervention with the outcomes that have been identified as the goals. Evidence-based practices from other disciplines and research need to be integrated into geriatric care management (e.g., depression interventions, fall prevention, dementia screening) to address specific problems and needs. Additionally, models of care management cannot be expected to address all problems for all populations, a 'one size fits all' solution that is doomed to fail. Specific protocols are needed that will include designated guidelines, time frames, contact schedules for follow-up and discrete, focused goals for the problem which it is attempting to address. Finally, outcomes measurement must act as a continual feedback loop, in which the information provided is easily available and useful to staff informing them of the effectiveness of their practice and ways in which they can better serve their target population.

As a result of the findings from this study, new models of care management were developed which addressed all of the issues listed above. These new programs incorporate the use of evidence-based clinical techniques, such as problem solving therapy, brief negotiation, and behavior change interventions, to empower patients to continually address and resolve issues that arise due to their health status. Preliminary findings from studies testing the efficacy of these new models improved outcomes in all the dependent variables measured in this study. More is not necessarily better in terms of services, resources, and benefits. Although clinicians did not anticipate the outcomes of this GCM evaluation the findings stimulated a shift in practice patterns. As a result, the use of evidence-based practice has contributed to the development of a learning culture with Kaiser and within the practice of social work.

REFERENCES

Boult, C., Rassen, J., Rassen, A., Moore, R., & Robison, S. (2000). The Effect of Case Management on the Costs of Health Care for Enrollees in Medicare Plus Choice Plans: A Randomized Trial. *Journal of the American Geriatrics Society, 4548*(8), 996-1001.

Brandt, T., Spencer, M., & Folstein, M. (1996). Telephone Interview for Cognitive Status. *Clinical Nursing Research, 5*, 185-198.

Breen, R. (1996). *Regression models: Censored, sample selected, or truncated data.* Thousand Oaks, CA: Sage Publications.

Brody, K. K., Johnson, R. E., & Ried, D. (1997). Evaluation of a Self-Report Screening Instrument to Predict Frailty Outcomes in Aging Populations. *The Gerontologist, 37*(2), 182-191.

Carter, D. (1996). Barriers to the implementation of research findings in practice. *Nurse Researcher, 4*(2), 30-40.

Claridge, J. A., & Fabian, T. C. (2005). History and Development of Evidence-based Medicine. *World J Surg*.

Engelhardt, J. B., Toseland, R. W., O'Donnell, J. C., Richie, J. T., Donald, J., & Banks, S. (1996). The Effectiveness and Efficiency of Outpatient Geriatric Evaluation and Management. *Journal of the American Geriatrics Society, 44*(7), 847-856.

Fordyce, M., Bardole, D., Romer, L., Soghikian, K., & Fireman, B. (1997). Senior Team Assessment and Referral Program-STAR. *The Journal of the American Board of Family Practice, 10*(6), 398-406.

Gagnon, A., Schein, C., McVey, L., & Bergman, H. (1999). Randomized Controlled Trial of Nurse Case Management of Frail Older People. *Journal of the American Geriatrics Society, 47*(9), 1118-11124.

Gallagher, D., Rappaport, M., Benedict, A., Lovett, S., & Silven, D. (1985). *Reliability of selected interview and self-report measures with family caregivers.* New Orleans: Gerontological Society of America.

Gorey, K. M. (1996). Effectiveness of social work intervention research: Internal versus external evaluations. *Social Work Research, 20*(2), 119-129.

Hassinger, M. (1985). *Community-dwelling dementia patients whose relatives sought counseling services regarding patient care: Predictors of institutionalization over a one-year follow-up period.* University of Southern California, Los Angeles.

IOM. (2001). *Crossing the Quality Chasm: A New Health System for the 21st Century.* Washington, D.C: National Academy Press.

Katz, S., & Akpom, C. (1976). A measure of primary sociobiological functions. *International Journal of Health Service, 6*, 496-507.

Lee, D., Mackenzie, A., Dudley-Brown, S., & Chin, T. M. (1998). Case Management: A Review of the Definitions and Practices. *Journal of Advanced Nursing, 27*(5), 933-939.

Leveille, S. G., Wagner, E. H., Davis, C., Grothaus, L., Wallace, J., LoGerfo, M. et al. (1998). Preventing disability and managing chronic illness in frail older adults: A randomized trial of a community-based partnership with primary care. [see comments.]. *Journal of the American Geriatrics Society, 46*(10), 1191-1198.

Long, M. J., & Marshall, B. S. (1999). Case management and the cost of care in the last month of life: Evidence from one managed care setting. *Health Care Manage Rev, 24*(4), 45-53.

Marshall, B. S., Long, M., Voss, J., Demma, K., & Skerl, K. P. (1999). Case Management of the Elderly in a Health Maintenance Organization: The Implications for Program Administration Under Managed Care. *Journal of Healthcare Management, 44*(6), 477-493.

Morishita, L., Boult, C., Boult, L., Smith, S., & Pacala, J. T. (1998). Satisfaction with Outpatient Geriatric Evaluation and Management (GEM). *The Gerontologist, 38*(3), 303-308.

Nalyor, M., Brooten, D., Campbell, R., Jacobsen, B. S., Mezey, M. D., Pauly, M. V. et al. (1999). Comprehensive Discharge Planning and Home Follow-up of Hospitalized Elders. *Journal of the American Medical Association, 281*(7), 613-620.

National Chronic Care Consortium (NCCC). (1997). *Case management for the frail elderly: A literature review on selected topics*: NCCC.

Orme, J. G., & Buehler, C. (2001). Introduction to multiple regression for categorical and limited dependent variables. *Social Work Research, 25*(1), 49-58.

Parker, G. (1997). Case Management: An Evidence-Based Review Fails to Make its Case. *Current Opinion in Psychiatry, 10*(4), 261-263.

Pryjmachuk, S. (1996). A nursing perspective on the interrelationships between theory, research and practice. *J Adv Nurs, 23*(4), 679-684.

Reid, W. J., Kenaley, B. D., Colvin, J., & Fortune, A. E. (2004). Do some interventions work better than others? A review of comparative social work experiments. *Social Work Research, 28*(2), p71, 11p.

Rosen, A., Proctor, E. K., & Staudt, M. M. (1999). Social work research and the quest for effective practice. *Social Work Research, 23*(1), p4, 11p.

Rosen, R. (2000). Applying research to health care policy and practice: Medical and managerial views on effectiveness and the role of research. *J Health Serv Res Policy, 5*(2), 103-108.

Schore, J. L., Brown, R. S., & Cheh, V. A. (1999). Case Management for High-Cost Medicare Beneficiaries. *Health Care Financing Review, 20*(4), 87-100.

Teri, L., Truax, P., Logsdon, R., Uomoto, J., Zarit, S. H., & Vitaliano, P. (1992). Assessment of Behavioral Problems in Dementia: The Revised Memory and Behavior Problems Checklist. *Psychology & Aging, 7*(4), 622-631.

Trella, R. (1993). A Multidisciplinary Approach to Case Management of Frail, Hospitalized Older Adults. *JONA, 23*(2), 20-26.

Weuve, J. L., Boult, C., & Morishita, L. (2000). The Effect of Outpatient Geriatric Evaluation and Management on Caregiver Burden. *The Gerontologist, 40*(4), 429-436.

Zarit, S. H., & Zarit, J. M. (1983). *The Memory and Behavior Problems Checklist and the Burden Interview*. University Park: Penn State Gerontology Center.

Implications
of Translating Research into Practice:
A Medication Management Intervention

Gretchen E. Alkema, MSW, LCSW
Dennee Frey, PharmD

SUMMARY. Through programs such as the Administration on Aging's Evidence-Based Prevention Initiative, researchers and practitioners are developing translational research studies seeking to implement rigorously tested, evidence-based interventions in new practice settings and evaluate the continuing effectiveness of these interventions. One such translational study is the Community-Based Medications Management Intervention (CBM Intervention), a collaborative effort to implement a medication management screening and intervention protocol in community-based waiver care management programs. The overall goals of the CBM Intervention are to implement an evidence-based medication management intervention in a California Medicaid waiver care management program, and to evaluate the effect of client-, intervention-, and organizational-level characteristics on resolving identified medication problems.

This article presents the need for improved medication management in a

---

Gretchen E. Alkema is affiliated with the Leonard Davis School of Gerontology, University of Southern California. Dennee Frey is affiliated with the Partners in Care Foundation.

The project described in this article was supported by a grant from the Administration on Aging (AoA) Evidence-Based Prevention Initiative.

[Haworth co-indexing entry note]: "Implications of Translating Research into Practice: A Medication Management Intervention." Alkema, Gretchen E., and Dennee Frey. Co-published simultaneously in *Home Health Care Services Quarterly* (The Haworth Press, Inc.) Vol. 25, No. 1/2, 2006, pp. 33-54; and: *Evidence-Based Interventions for Community Dwelling Older Adults* (ed: Susan M. Enguídanos) The Haworth Press, Inc., 2006, pp. 33-54. Single or multiple copies of this article are available for a fee from The Haworth Document Delivery Service [1-800-HAWORTH, 9:00 a.m. - 5:00 p.m. (EST). E-mail address: docdelivery@ haworthpress.com].

33

frail, community-dwelling, older adult population and describes the CBM Intervention as an example of translating an evidence-based practice beyond its original efficacy trial in a home healthcare program into a care management program. It discusses critical factors involved in translating research into practice using a translational research framework, Promoting Action on Research Implementation in Health Services (PARIHS). Our experience suggests that although implementing research into practice can positively impact client care, professional skill enhancement and organizational effectiveness, this is very challenging work requiring signification facilitation for successful outcomes. *[Article copies available for a fee from The Haworth Document Delivery Service: 1-800-HAWORTH. E-mail address: <docdelivery@haworthpress.com> Website: <http://www.HaworthPress.com> © 2006 by The Haworth Press, Inc. All rights reserved.]*

KEYWORDS. Evidence-based, translational research, older adults, care management program, medication management, medication-related problems

INTRODUCTION

Health services professionals have long recognized the importance of integrating research and practice to improve quality of care and health-related quality of life. Over the last several decades, researchers and practitioners have joined forces to develop translational research studies that seek to implement rigorously tested, evidence-based interventions in new practice settings and evaluate the continuing effectiveness of these interventions. One such translational study is the Community- Based Medications Management Intervention (CBM Intervention), a collaborative effort to implement a medication management screening and intervention protocol in community-based care management programs. The overall goals of the Community-Based Medications Management Intervention are to implement an evidence-based medication management intervention in a Medicaid waiver care management program operating in two different agencies, and to evaluate its impact on reducing medication problems for frail older adults.

In September 2003, the CBM Intervention was launched as part of the Administration on Aging's Evidence-Based Disease Prevention Initiative. This three-year initiative was developed to support the implementation of evidence-based practice at the community level through the aging service provider network. Each of the thirteen funded projects is implementing an intervention initially tested in a randomized control trial environment and found to be effective in promoting disease prevention with community-dwelling older adults, often with multiple and complex needs.

Evidence for the success of this medication management model intervention comes from a multi-site, multi-phase study conducted by Vanderbilt University researchers in a home health care setting. Among study findings is that the prevalence of medication-related problems or potential errors ranged from 17 up to 30% using study and other criteria. In a randomized control trial the home healthcare-based intervention reduced medication problems between 12% and 47% in a sample of community-dwelling Medicare-beneficiaries aged 65 and older (Meredith et al., 2002). Building on this work, this article will (1) detail the need for medication management in the older adult population, (2) discuss challenges to implementing research into practice, and (3) describe the Community-Based Medication Management Intervention as an example of translating an evidence-based practice beyond its original efficacy trial in Medicare-certified home healthcare agency setting to a community-based waiver care management program. Given the multiplicity of factors involved in translating research into practice, a translational research framework, Promoting Action on Research Implementation in Health Services (PARIHS) (Kitson et al., 1998; Rycroft-Malone, Harvey et al., 2004; Rycroft-Malone et al., 2002), is used to organize and clarify critical translational factors.

THE NEED FOR MEDICATION MANAGEMENT

Although older adults represent only 13% of the United States population, they consume over one-third of all prescription drugs (Families USA, 2000; Kahl et al., 1992). Nearly half of those aged 65 and over report taking three or more medications on a monthly basis, compared to just over one-third ten years ago (National Center for Health Statistics, 2004). Sixty-two percent of older adults have two or more chronic conditions (Wu & Green, 2000), further increasing the chances of multiple physicians prescribing multiple medications. Inappropriate medication use by adults living independently in the community has been reported to range from 12 to 40% (Zhan et al., 2001). Adverse drug events, defined as an injury due to an adverse drug reaction or a medication error (Silverman et al., 2004), directly account for 7,000 deaths each year (Institute of Medicine, 2000; Phillips et al., 1998). Nationwide, the average cost of medication-related problems and their associated conditions is over $2 billion annually and is expected to increase as more medications enter the marketplace with unknown interaction effects with existing prescription drugs (Institute of Medicine, 2000). A recent study reports that over one-quarter of adverse drug events in ambulatory settings are preventable (Gurwitz et al., 2003).

Several studies point to human and system-level errors as contributing factors to medication problems and their associated results (Aparasu & Sitzman, 1999; Coleman, 2003; Curtis et al., 2004; Fu et al., 2004; Goulding, 2004; Howard et al., 2004; Institute of Medicine, 2000). These studies call for changes in prescribing patterns and increased use of decision support tools to reduce inappropriate prescribing. A recent survey of health care experts reported that improving the quality and safety of medical care by expanding the use of technology is a top health policy priority, second only to expanded healthcare coverage to the uninsured (The Commonwealth Fund, 2004). One promising intervention, medication management, includes medication screening at multiple phases in the pharmaceutical process and the implementation of change strategies to ameliorate identified problems using human and/or computerized technology. Technologies generally used to support medication management include computerized physician order entry, automated dispensing in institutional settings, and drug utilization review systems. Prior research has evaluated the implementation of medication management processes using human (Gilbert et al., 2002) or technological (Glassman et al., 2002; Tamblyn et al., 2003) methods alone in multiple health care settings. However, the most powerful interventions appear to be those that incorporate human review with technology and evidence-based guidelines as decisional support mechanisms (Monane et al., 1998; Silverman et al., 2004). For older adults prescribed multiple drugs, medication review technology that assists health care providers with decisional support offers an effective and efficient means to address medication problems (Gurwitz et al., 2003).

CHALLENGES AND OPPORTUNITIES FOR TRANSLATIONAL RESEARCH

Several health care agencies and initiatives have called for improved strategies to address medication-related problems (Clancy et al., 2004;

Institute of Medicine, 2001; Quality Interagency Coordination Task Force, 2000; The Commonwealth Fund, 2004) (Department of Health and Human Services, 2000) (Clancy, 2004). In this context, researchers must take the lead by working collaboratively with practitioners to develop and translate evidence-based practices that meet the needs of consumers, providers, and health and long-term care systems. However, to date there has been very little translation of evidence-based practice into community agencies (Bellg et al., 2004; Feldman & Kane, 2003).

Translating evidence-based practice into community agencies has the potential to drastically improve treatment effectiveness and reduce provider variability in applying treatment regimens (Feldman & Kane, 2003). Moreover, community services agencies, which often have less external oversight than health care models, can demonstrate improved quality of care by implementing tested interventions rather than building their own models, which may leave out important components (Institute of Medicine, 2001). The use of empirically tested interventions also promotes cost effectiveness for community-based agencies by focusing on efficacious interventions known to work with targeted problems and populations (Weissert et al., 2003). However, there are multiple challenges to translating evidence-based practices into community settings including: resistance to practice modalities by professionals; lack of organizational buy-in; lack of specific goals and standards in translating the evidence; and rigidity of evidence-based practice that cannot be molded to meet specific needs of the applied setting (Glasgow et al., 2003; Grimshaw et al., 2001; Grol, 2001).

A critical feature to translating research into practice is the need to resolve the tension between treatment fidelity and reasonable adaptation to the implementing program (Backer, 2001). When implementing evidence-based research into "real-life" programs, some researchers believe that treatment protocols created in a research environment must be strictly adhered to in order for the new iteration to be accurately described as a "true" adopter (Bellg et al., 2004; Elliott & Mihalic, 2004; Titler, 2004). Some argue that the lack of evidence-based practice in community service programs ultimately devalues social services in the eyes of other more medically focused professions that socialize their practitioners toward the benefit of standardized practice regimens (Murphy & McDonald, 2004). Others note that treatment fidelity purists focus so much on the technicalities of implementing the evidence-based practice that key characteristics of the adopting agency and target population are disregarded, often leading to implementation failure (Castro et al., 2004; Dusenbury & Hansen,

2004; Leventhal & Friedman, 2004). Given these inherent tensions, the Community-Based Medication Management Intervention hopes to move beyond an "all or nothing" approach to translational research by identifying the key factors critical to the translation process as well as those factors that may be adapted to promote successful implementation in new settings.

DIFFUSION OF EVIDENCE-BASED PRACTICES

A variety of disciplines have examined the process of diffusing innovative practices into applied settings (Bradley et al., 2004; Glasgow et al., 2003; Glasgow et al., 2001; Glasgow et al., 1999; National Center for HIV Prevention, 2003; Rogers, 1995; Rycroft-Malone, Harvey et al., 2004; Walshe & Rundall, 2001). Although originating from different fields, researchers from these studies all suggest the importance of three basic elements in translating evidence-based practices: (1) the qualities and characteristics of the evidence being implemented; (2) the organizational and social system that will be accepting the new evidence; and (3) the various communication processes by which the evidence is sown and takes root in the new setting. However, much of the previous work remains atheoretical, leaving researchers with little guidance to systematically monitor implementation of innovations into novel settings. One translational paradigm, the PARIHS (the Promoting Action on Research Implementation in Health Services) framework (Kitson et al., 1998; Rycroft-Malone, Harvey et al., 2004; Rycroft-Malone et al., 2002), does offer a structured mechanism to understand the complexities of translating research into practice.

The PARIHS framework describes three constructs that are critical in understanding how research-tested intervention strategies are successfully implemented into practice settings: (1) evidence (Rycroft-Malone, Seers et al., 2004), (2) context (McCormack et al., 2002), and (3) facilitation (Harvey et al., 2002). Evidence includes scientifically robust data, protocols, or other intervention material that will be implemented in a site as well as professional experience and consumer preferences within the site that will impact implementation (Rycroft-Malone, Seers et al., 2004). Context includes the physical, social, professional, cultural, and leadership environment in which the evidence will be adopted (McCormack et al., 2002). Facilitation addresses the management and administrative attributes of the implementing site that will support and assist implementation of the evidence into the context (Harvey et al., 2002). Each of these constructs has several characteristics to further describe the underlying mechanisms (see Rycroft-Malone et al. (2002) for more detail).

Developers of the PARIHS framework hypothesize that successful implementation will occur when: (1) the evidence is scientifically robust, matching professional consensus and client needs ("high evidence"); (2) the context is receptive to change with strong leadership and appropriate monitoring and feedback systems ("high context"); and (3) there is appropriate facilitation of change with input from skilled internal and external facilitators ("high facilitation") (Kitson et al., 1998; Rycroft-Malone et al., 2002). Although the PARIHS framework clearly does not include all potential variables that may impact the implementation process, it is an orienting perspective that can shed light on the complex world of translating research into practice. We use this framework to delineate characteristic differences at two levels of the translational process: First, differences between the original randomized control trial in home healthcare agencies and the new MSSP care management sites; and second, among the multiple MSSP sites implementing the evidence-based medication management intervention.

EVIDENCE-BASED PRACTICE: THE HOME HEALTH CRITERIA AND MEDICATION MANAGEMENT MODEL INTERVENTION

The evidence-based practice model employed in the current CBM Intervention originated in a home healthcare setting (Brown et al., 1998), empirically tested by Vanderbilt University researchers through a randomized control trial design (Meredith et al., 2002; Meredith et al., 2001). An expert consensus panel initially developed the Home Health Criteria (HH Criteria), to identify home healthcare patients whose patterns of medication use, combined with clinical signs and symptoms, indicated potential risk for potential adverse events. These criteria focus on factors that can be assessed most easily by home health nurses and resolved as part of a home health plan of care (Brown et al., 1998).

The four categories of medication problems comprising the Home Health Criteria are:

1. Inappropriate therapeutic duplication of medications;

2. Cardiovascular medication problems, e.g., uncontrolled hypertension;
3. Inappropriate psychotropic medication use with concurrent falls or confusion; and
4. Inappropriate use of non-steroidal anti-inflammatory drugs.

Data used to determine a potential medication problem were the patient's current medication list, age, and functional information from the home healthcare nursing assessment. Functional data assessed were the following five evidence-based clinical indicators that related specifically to the defined medication problems in an attempt to reduce false positive screening errors: blood pressure, pulse rate, recent falls, confusion, and dizziness.

To determine the frequency of medication problems in the home healthcare population, Vanderbilt researchers studied and compared the HH Criteria and the Beers Criteria, which is widely used to identify potentially inappropriate medication use by the elderly (Beers, 1997). Based on the HH Criteria, Vanderbilt researchers reported initial prevalence data that 19% of the home healthcare sample (N = 6,718) had at least one medication problem as compared to 17% using the Beers criteria (Meredith et al., 2001). Prevalence rates using either of the home healthcare screening criteria or the Beers were comparable, yet when both criteria were used, medication problem rates increased to 30% of the sample. Additionally, over 30% of those in the sample who had at least one medication problem (N = 1,279) were taking nine or more medications daily (Meredith et al., 2001). These prevalence data speak to the vulnerability of older adults to medication problems and raise great concern about potential adverse consequences.

Building on these results, Vanderbilt researchers and clinical co-investigators developed a medication use improvement program called the Medication Management Model (MMM). The goal of MMM is to address medication problems identified in this sample and beyond using both human and technological capacities. The intervention centered on the role of a consultant pharmacist within the home healthcare setting to assist nursing staff with identifying, preventing, and resolving medication problems among community-dwelling, high-risk older adults. Two large home healthcare agency sites piloted this medication management intervention using a randomized control trial design to evaluate its efficacy in this setting.

Below are the core elements of MMM as tested in the home healthcare randomized control trial:

- A computerized screening algorithm identified patients who had one of four medication problems according to the HH Criteria.
- Those with a verified medication problem were included in the study and randomly assigned to intervention and control conditions.
- A structured in-home assessment was conducted by a trained research assistant to verify problem and obtain informed consent.
- Once verified, the pharmacist was alerted of the intervention patients.
- The pharmacist and nurse assessed the patients' data using study medication improvement protocols to verify the problem and to develop recommendations.
- The nurse contacted the prescribing physician to alert him/her to the specific medication problem using a structured template for discussion
- For complex cases (e.g., cases involving tapering of psychotropic medications), the pharmacist contacted the physician directly regarding suggested medication changes;
- Nurse informed the patient of the medication issue, assisted with medication changes, and monitored effects of the medication change; and
- Control subjects received usual and customary services from home healthcare nurses.
- A research assistant collected outcome data for all study participants within 90 days.

Utilizing this approach, medication problems were resolved for 50% of intervention group (N = 130), compared to 38% in the control group (N = 129; p < .05) (Meredith et al., 2002). Intervention participants who had therapeutic duplication as their medication problem showed a 71% reduction in medication problems after the intervention (N = 17), compared to 24% in the control group (N = 24; p < .003) (Meredith et al., 2002). Use of cardiovascular medications also improved with a 37% reduction of problems for the intervention group (Meredith et al., 2002).

In a third phase of the project, technical assistance was provided to four additional home healthcare agencies of varying characteristics interested in adapting what is now the Medication Management Model into everyday practice. Among the lessons learned was that the model is feasible, flexible, and sustainable, and the intervention may be applicable to other programs providing in-home services to frail older adults (Frey & Rahman, 2003).

TRANSLATING THE MEDICATION MANAGEMENT MODEL INTO NEW SETTINGS

Upon demonstrated efficacy of the medication management intervention, developers focused on translating the intervention beyond the Medicare-certified home healthcare setting to a wider practice audience serving populations at high risk for medication problems. In this vein, the CBM Intervention is translating the MMM based on the original program design into a care management program that serves disabled, multi-ethnic, low-income older adults living in the community–the Multipurpose Senior Service Program (MSSP). MSSP is a California Medicaid waiver program that provides care management and purchase of services to eligible low-income older adults in an effort to decrease inappropriate institutionalization. MSSP clients are community-dwelling adults aged 65 and over who are Medicaid eligible, and demonstrate significant functional impairment as evidenced by (1) two or more activities of daily living impairments or (2) at least one activity of daily living deficiency and cognitive impairment. All newly enrolled and existing MSSP clients from the participating programs are screened for medication problems using a risk-screening algorithm developed by the original researchers and based on the original screening algorithm. For new clients, the intervention process begins upon initial assessment; continuing clients begin the intervention process at the 6-month or annual re-assessment visit, whichever comes first.

Two community-based agencies in Southern California that operate the MSSP care management program are participating in the CBM Intervention. MSSP A is implementing the medication management intervention first in two sites, Burbank (Site #1) and Lynwood (Site #2); Site #1 piloted the medication management intervention first with Site #2 following three months later. In April 2005, MSSP B (Site #3 in Pasadena) begins implementation. It is anticipated that the Site #3 will benefit from lessons learned at the first two sites in dealing with context and facilitation challenges.

Figure 1 describes the translation process through the adopting agencies, starting with the MSSP A sites as the initial adopting agency that is guiding the MSSP B through implementation. By using care management systems as the vehicle for a first-generation implementation study, the CBM Intervention is expanding the vision of the intervention and testing the boundary tension between model fidelity and adaptation to a "real world" practice environment (Castro et al., 2004; Elliott & Mihalic, 2004) that serves disabled, low-income, culturally diverse older adults.

FIGURE 1. Translational Design for the Community-Based Medications Management Intervention Project

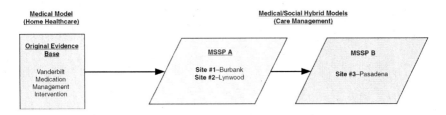

DESCRIPTION OF IMPLEMENTATION IN CARE MANAGEMENT

The implementation of the MMM in the MSSP care management sites follows a nearly identical process as in the original home healthcare setting. This process is described below and represented graphically in Figure 2.

- Nurse and social worker care managers complete usual assessments that include a current list of medication and five clinical indicators (blood pressure, pulse, recent falls, confusion, and dizziness) deemed relevant from the original study;
- Data are entered into existing agency database that includes computerized medication risk assessment screening algorithm based on the original algorithm;
- Based on usual practice, client is randomly assigned to a primary care manager–either the nurse or social worker;
- Pharmacist reviews cases with computerized alerts to validate medication problem (Prevalence in Figure 2 below) or identifies potential problems via manual screening;
- Pharmacist discuss cases with primary care manager and to develop care plans and determine follow-up responsibility using protocols from the original study;
- Primary care manager contacts prescribing physician to inform of the medication problem based on above (Time 1);
- In complex medication cases, pharmacist contacts the prescribing physician, providing alternative medication recommendations. Communications are in writing and transmitted via fax to physician's office;

- Primary care manager educates client/caregiver about the identified medication problems, and discusses ways to improve health status related to the specific problem; and
- Primary care manager follows up with client with identified problems at three-month visit and inquires about medication changes (Time 2).

IMPLEMENTATION IN A DIFFERENT PROGRAM

As a translational research issue, there are similarities and differences between the CBM Intervention Project sites (MSSP) and the original home healthcare randomized control trial. Some apparent similarities across sites include:

- Client population of high-risk community dwelling older adults with co-morbid medical conditions
- Community-based settings serving diverse geographic areas and racial/ethnic compositions of clients
- Reliance on government funding streams
- Strict regulatory environment

However, differences between the original trial and the first-generation implementation are uniquely relevant in terms of how it impacts the balance between intervention fidelity and adaptation. These organizational variables are relevant in assessing the overall feasibility of translating the Medication Management Model intervention into the applied practice settings. Differences between the home health randomized

FIGURE 2. Implementation of the Community-Based Medication Management Intervention

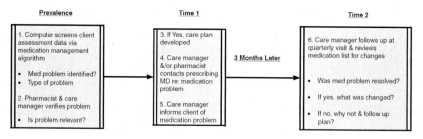

control trial environment and the translation sites using the PARIHS framework are listed in Table 1.

As described above, the MSSP care management program differs in several ways from the original home healthcare program in the randomized trial. Nationwide, Medicare-certified home healthcare programs operate as short-term medical model programs requiring physician orders and oversight. Patients admitted to home healthcare often are recently discharged from a hospital setting following an acute illness and need skilled nursing care at home with Medicare as the primary payer of service. Conversely, the California waiver care management programs provide long-term care and support services for their clients using a medical/social hybrid model approach of quarterly in-home assessment visits and monthly telephone follow-up. Additionally, the care management program serves adults aged 65 and above who are low-income, disabled, chronically ill, racially and ethnically diverse, and community-dwelling with nearly all qualifying as dually eligible for Medicare and Medicaid services.

COMPARISONS OF MSSP PROGRAM SITES

Similarities of sites within the two organizations include a decidedly functionally-impaired client population, basic staffing requirements for social workers (2/3) and registered nurses (1/3), structured procedures for client visitation and documentation, and Medicaid funding. However, each site has unique characteristics in terms of operational style and programmatic engagement with clients, creating another layer of complexity to the translation of the medications management intervention. Table 2 clarifies these differences below.

Sites #1 and #3 utilize both nurses and social workers as primary care managers, whereas Site #2 employs nurses in a consultative role. Clients in Sites #1 and #3 are randomly assigned to the care manager type, but both a nurse and social worker complete independent assessments of the client upon initial enrollment. In contrast, nurses in Site #2 complete their initial assessment upon enrollment, but do not carry an ongoing caseload. Therefore, nurses in Site #2 might be less likely to contact the prescribing physician in the event of a medication problem. This situation means that social workers in Site #2, who generally operate from a more social model approach to treatment, will be expected to discuss the medication problem that is a medically related issue with the prescribing physician.

TABLE 1. Differences Between Home Healthcare and MSSP Programs

	Original MMM trial in Home Health	Translational Sites in MSSP
Evidence		
# of participants	N = 259	Capacity: 1,235
Inclusion criteria for translation	Likelihood of survival; client to understand spoken English	Community-dwelling; No language requirement
Core element of intervention	Intervention a structured collaboration between clinical pharmacist and RN employing medication improvement protocols	Intervention a collaboration among Pharm and CMs (RN or SW) guided by updated protocols
Medication Management Model protocols and expected variation	• Study computerized screening algorithm alerts for problems in intervention clients and verified by research assistant • Pharm reviewed medications for intervention clients • Pharm informed RN of problem and formulated care plan using protocols; RN contacts MD and fulfilled next steps • If changes needed, RNs helped with medication changes and educated client • Pharm discussed complicated medication problems with MDs and provided education materials to RNs	• Created risk assessment screening and medication database using Home Health algorithm • Database alerts Pharm, who reviews w/CM using updated protocols based on Home Health Criteria • CM contacts MD re: medication problem • If med changes needed, CM informs client about problem • Pharm contacts MD re: complicated problems; change in orders relayed to CM and client
Enrollment requirements of program	• Admission to home healthcare service requires MD orders	• Enrollment by client choice and does not require MD orders
Pre and post measurements	Pre–Initial assessment Post–6 weeks to 90 days after initial assessment	Pre–initial assessment Post–at 3 month quarterly visit after initial assessment
Measures used beyond the scope of standard practice	Randomized controlled trial Measured: SF-36 Mini-Mental ADL total dependence	Mini-mental status completed by both RN & SW care managers Reassessment includes evidence-based clinical indicators
Context		
Organizational philosophy	Medical Model program	Medical/social hybrid model program
Estimated client length of stay	4 weeks	Ranges from 1 month to years
Staff participation in intervention	HHA nurses (RNs) and Pharm	Care managers (RNs & Master's level SWs) & Pharm
Staff visitation	Several times a week	Monthly phone calls and quarterly visits
Documentation methods	RN progress notes, Pharm consultation/progress notes, and intervention summary sheets	MSSP sites–Computerized records (assessment, reassessment and progress notes for CMs & Pharm consultation/progress notes)
Facilitation		
Training associated with Home Health Model	1-2 sessions–approximately 3-4 hrs total	1 orientation and at least 1 clinical session per site. Additional training planned to reinforce Home Health Model

Facilitation (continued)		
Facilitation monitoring	Site visits to monitor progress. Minimal process follow-up with staff. Some with administrators & consultant pharmacists	Process evaluation with staff before & after implementation; staff involved in process Evaluators monitoring phase-in meetings & ongoing implementation at sites
Types of partners assisting in this project and their roles	• Vanderbilt Researchers • Home Health Agency Program Directors/managers in 2 sites • Consensus Panel of experts developed Home Health Criteria • Medical consultation provided by clinical pharmacologist (N. Brown, MD, VU) • Home Health Advisory panel for technical assistance/dissemination phase	• Original co-investigator is Project Director • Original expert panel member • Geriatric Advisory; Original advisory panel member. On-going medical and protocol consultation provided by advisors • Local hospital medical staff as healthcare partner • MSSP software developer to create screening tool • Local university evaluation researcher

Legend:
CM = Care managers
HHA = Home Healthcare Agency nurses
MSSP = Multipurpose Senior Services Program
MD = Prescribing medical doctor
MMM = Medication Management Model
Pharm = Consultant pharmacist
RN = Registered nurses
SW = Social workers

TABLE 2. Context and Facilitation Differences Between MSSP Care Management Sites

Total N = 1,235	Site #1 (Burbank; N = 206)	Site #2 (Lynwood; N = 566)	Site #3 (Pasadena; N = 463)
Context			
Care manager role	Nurses & social workers as primary care managers	Social workers as primary care managers; nurses as consultants	Nurses & social workers as primary care managers
Presence of consulting Pharmacist	Pharmacist regularly on site and by phone occasionally	Pharmacist available by phone and occasionally on site	Pharmacist available by phone and occasionally on site
Site Management	MSSP A	MSSP A	MSSP B
Facilitation			
Facilitation process	Project lead and first implementation site	Second implementation site	Third implementation site
Presence of facilitation team	Team housed at site	Team on site for meetings and has phone consults	Team on site for meetings and has phone consults

Legend:
N = MSSP program capacity

In addition, Site #2 will not have the benefit of regular face-to-face contact with the consultant pharmacist to address medication questions as they arise. This arrangement may have an impact on the implementation of the intervention, as described further in the hypotheses below. Care managers at Site #1 also have the opportunity for daily contact with the project facilitation team and are the first site to implement the intervention. A further organizational difference is that MSSP #A (Sites #1 and #2) are independent of a medical setting, but MSSP #B (Site #3) is affiliated with and on-site at a local hospital. This proximity to health care services, both organizationally and geographically, may also impact the staff's ability to implement the medication management intervention.

EVALUATION PLAN

As evidence-based interventions are transplanted into applied settings, it is important to evaluate both the effectiveness of the intervention in the new sites as well as understanding the process of implementing (Rossi et al., 2004; Weiss, 1997; Wholey et al., 2004). In this light, the CBM Intervention includes a program evaluation in the overall implementation design in order to (1) understand the progression and impact of translating evidence-based practices into new and different community settings, and (2) to evaluate the benefits and challenges of translating the Medication Management Intervention into practice for first-generation adopters outside of the medical model environment. This evaluation is analyzing the intended outcomes of reducing medication problems in a sample of frail, community-dwelling older adults. Additionally, it includes a process evaluation to capture both implementation fidelity and changes to the intervention as needed by the unique MSSP operational environment.

Outcomes Evaluation

The outcomes evaluation will appraise the translation of the evidence-based medication management intervention from a medical model home healthcare program into a medical/social hybrid model care management program focusing on its ability to identify and reduce medication problems for MSSP clients. To determine frequency and extent of identifying and reducing medication problems for MSSP clients, the specific aims of the outcome evaluation are to:

1. Describe prevalence rates of medication problems identified in three MSSP sites; and
2. Identify client outcomes of implementing the medication management intervention in the MSSP sites including:

   a. Rates of resolving identified medication problems; and
   b. The effect of client-, intervention-, and organizational-level characteristics on resolving identified medication problems.

Process Evaluation

The process evaluation will focus on implementation fidelity of translating the Home Health Model into the MSSP sites, inquiring about the extent to which sites adhered to the Home Health Model during implementation. If the sites demonstrate departures from the Home Health Model, the evaluation will explore how these factors affected the implementation process and ultimately client outcomes. Given the possibility that the MMM conceived in the home healthcare setting will require revision at some level to function in a care management environment, the process evaluation will examine what factors in the intervention have changed to fit into the new practice settings (the key characteristics), and what factors have remained constant throughout the intervention (the core elements) (National Center for HIV Prevention, 2003).

Qualitative methods will be used to complete the process evaluation outlined for this study including (1) reviewing and analyzing focus group transcripts with staff and program administrators, and (2) participant-observer methods at implementation training sessions, staff meetings, and advisory group meetings (Weiss, 1997). Focus groups with staff program directors will inquire about their perceptions of implementation using the PARIHS constructs of context, evidence, and facilitation as a guide. Participant-observer methods have already been used in initial training sessions with MSSP #1 staff and advisory group meetings. This method was vitally useful in understanding the differences between the original and implementation sites. Future participation in these meetings will build on this experience and is anticipated to reveal the essence of the translational process beyond the program's outcomes.

CONCLUSION

The Community-Based Medication Management Intervention brings several strengths and faces some challenges in translating an evidence-based practice into existing programs. Strengths include a unique and current data source from an established long-term care program, a highly diverse sample of frail older adults, and the participation of two well-respected organizations committed to improving medication safety for this population. The lead organization is following the evidence-based practice approach described by Altpeter et al. (2006) in considering important risk factors and health conditions in the target population selected. Evidence-based program planning and implementation activities that create the bridge between intervention research and practice are being evaluated and monitored by the evaluation partners. Strong partnerships with other MSSP organizations throughout the state and with national aging organizations will assist in the dissemination of findings and lessons learned. Data are also reflective of real-life practice and will provide insight into the process and outcomes of translating evidence-based interventions into applied settings.

Challenges faced in this process include (1) geographically and culturally diverse settings for implementation; (2) educational and training differences among staff; and (3) operational differences across the implementing sites. These factors suggest that although implementing research into practice is a valuable exercise positively impacting client care, professional skill enhancement and organizational effectiveness, this is still hard work requiring signification facilitation for successful outcomes.

The CBM Intervention exemplifies the translation of an evidence-based practice beyond its original efficacy trial in home healthcare sites to a different long-term care practice environment in the MSSP care management program. Although core features of original study are in effect to maintain fidelity to the evidence-based practice, minor modifications have been made to adapt the Medication Management Model to pre-existing contextual elements of the care management program and might affect the success of the intervention. Contextual differences include (1) the medical nature of home healthcare agency operations as opposed to the medical/social hybrid nature of MSSP programs; (2) perceived roles of different care management professions in medication management; (3) the brokerage nature of care management services intervention in MSSP. Additionally a primary facilitation issue is the variation in implementation process among the participating sites and across the two participating agencies.

To capture the breadth and depth of this translational project, the program evaluation not only will measure medication resolution outcomes on a client level, but also provide lessons learned on implementing an evidence-based practice in each MSSP site and care management programs overall. Given that MSSP clients are frail older adults at high risk for nursing home placement, reducing adverse drug events for this population through a systematic process of medication management is extremely critical to their overall health and quality of life and ability to maintain living in the community.

REFERENCES

Altpeter, M., Bryant L., Schneider, E., & Whitelaw, N. (2006). Evidence-based health practice: Knowing and using what works for older adults. *Home Health Care Services Quarterly, 25* (1&2), 1-11.

Aparasu, R. R., & Sitzman, S. J. (1999). Inappropriate prescribing for elderly outpatients. *American Journal of Health-System Pharmacy, 56*(5), 433-439.

Backer, T. E. (2001). Finding the Balance: Program Fidelity and Adaptation in Substance Abuse Prevention. Rockville, MD: Center for Substance Abuse Prevention.

Beers, M. H. (1997). Explicit criteria for determining potentially inappropriate medication use by the elderly. *Archives of Internal Medicine, 157*, 1531-1536.

Bellg, A. J., Borrelli, B., Barbara, R., Hecht, J., Minicucci, D. S., Ory, M., Ogedegbe, G., Orwig, D., Ernst, D., & Susan, C. (2004). Enhancing treatment fidelity in health behavior change studies: Best practices and recommendations from the NIH behavior change consortium. *Health Psychology, 23*(5), 443-451.

Bradley, E. H., Webster, T. R., Baker, D., Schlesinger, M., Inouye, S. K., Barth, M. C., Lapane, K. L., Lipson, D., Stone, R., & Koren, M. J. (2004). Translating research into practice: Speeding the adoption of innovative health care programs. New York: The Commonwealth Fund.

Brown, N. J., Griffin, M. R., Ray, W. A., Meredith, S., Beers, M. H., Marren, J., Robles, M., Stergachis, A., Wood, A. J., & Avorn, J. (1998). A model for improving medication use in home health care patients. *Journal of the American Pharmaceutical Association, 38*(6), 696-702.

Castro, F., Barrera, M., & Martinez, C. (2004). The cultural adaptation of prevention intervention: Resolving tensions between fidelity and fit. *Prevention Science, 5*(1), 41-45.

Clancy, C. M. (2004). AHRQ's FY 2005 budget request: New mission, new vision. *Health Services Research, 39*(3), xi-xviii.

Clancy, C. M., Slutsky, J. R., & Patton, L. T. (2004). Evidence-based health care 2004: AHRQ moves research to translation and implementation. *Health Services Research, 39*(5), xv-xxiii.

Coleman, E. A. (2003). Falling Through the Cracks: Challenges and Opportunities for Improving Transitional Care for Persons with Continuous Complex Care Needs. *Journal of the American Geriatrics Society, 51*(4), 549-555.

Curtis, L. H., Ostbye, T., Sendersky, V., Hutchison, S., Dans, P. E., Wright, A., Woosley, R. L., & Schulman, K. A. (2004). Inappropriate prescribing for elderly Americans in a large outpatient population. *Archives of Internal Medicine, 9*(23), 1621-1625.

Department of Health and Human Services. (2000). Healthy People 2010 (Objective 17.3). Washington, DC.

Dusenbury, L., & Hansen, W. B. (2004). Pursuing the course from research to practice. *Prevention Science, 5*(1), 55-59.

Elliott, D. S., & Mihalic, S. (2004). Issues in disseminating and replicating effective prevention programs. *Prevention Science, 5*(1), 47-53.

Families USA. (2000). Cost Overdose: Growth in Drug Spending for the Elderly, 1992-2010. Washington, DC.

Feldman, P. H., & Kane, R. L. (2003). Strengthening research to improve the practice and management of long-term care. *Milbank Quarterly, 81*(2), 179-220.

Frey, D., & Rahman, A. (2003). Medication management: An evidence-based model that decreases adverse events. *Home Healthcare Nurse, 21*(6), 404-412.

Fu, A. Z., Liu, G. G., & Christensen, D. B. (2004). Inappropriate medication use and health outcomes in the elderly. *Journal of the American Geriatrics Society, 52*(11), 1934-1939.

Gilbert, A. L., Roughead, E. E., Beilby, J., Mott, K., & Barratt, J. D. (2002). Collaborative medication management services: Improving patient care. *Medical Journal of Australia, 177*(4), 189-192.

Glasgow, R. E., Lichtenstein, E. P., & Marcus, A. C. (2003). Why don't we see more translation of health promotion research to practice? Rethinking the efficacy-to-effectiveness transition. *American Journal of Public Health, 93*(8), 1261-1267.

Glasgow, R. E., Orleans, C. T., & Wagner, E. H. (2001). Does the chronic care model serve also as a template for improving prevention? *Milbank Quarterly, 79*(4), 579-612.

Glasgow, R. E., Vogt, T. M., & Boles, S. M. (1999). Evaluating the Public Health Impact of Health Promotion Interventions: The RE-AIM Framework. *American Journal of Public Health September, 89*(9), 1322-1327.

Glassman, P. A., Simon, B., Belperio, P., & Lanto, A. (2002). Improving recognition of drug interactions: Benefits and barriers to using automated drug alerts. *Medical Care, 40*(12), 1161-1171.

Goulding, M. R. (2004). Inappropriate medication prescribing for elderly ambulatory care patients. *Archives of Internal Medicine, 164*(3), 305-312.

Grimshaw, J. M., Shirran, L., Thomas, R., Mowatt, G., Fraser, C., Bero, L., Grilli, R., Harvey, E., Oxman, A., & O'Brien, M. A. (2001). Changing provider behavior: An overview of systematic reviews of interventions. *Medical Care, 39*(8), II-2-II-45.

Grol, R. P. (2001). Successes and failures in the implementation of evidence-based guidelines for clinical practice. *Medical Care, 39*(8), II-46-II-54.

Gurwitz, J. H., Field, T. S., Harrold, L. R., Rothschild, J., Debellis, K., Seger, A. C., Cadoret, C., Fish, L. S., Garber, L., Kelleher, M., & Bates, D. W. (2003). Incidence and preventability of adverse drug events among older persons in the ambulatory setting. *Journal of the American Medical Association, 289*(9), 1107-1116.

Harvey, G., Loftus-Hills, A., Rycroft-Malone, J., Titchen, A., Kitson, A., McCormack, B., & Seers, K. (2002). Getting evidence into practice: The role and function of facilitation. *Journal of Advanced Nursing, 37*(6), 577-588.

Howard, M., Dolovich, L., Kaczorowski, J., Sellors, C., & Sellors, J. (2004). Prescribing of potentially inappropriate medications to elderly people. *Family Practice, 21*(3), 244-247.

Institute of Medicine. (2000). To err is human: Building a safer health system. Washington, D.C.: National Academy Press.

Institute of Medicine. (2001). Crossing the quality chasm: A new health system for the 21st century. Washington, D.C: National Academy Press.

Kahl, A., Blandford, D., Krueger, K., & Zwick, D. (1992). Geriatric education centers address medication issues affecting older adults. *Public Health Report, 107*(1), 37-47.

Kitson, A., Harvey, G., & McCormack, B. (1998). Enabling the implementation of evidence-based practice: A conceptual framework. *Quality in Health Care, 7,* 149-158.

Leventhal, H., & Friedman, M. A. (2004). Does establishing fidelity of treatment help in understanding treatment efficacy? Comment on Bellg et al. *Health Psychology, 23*(5), 452-456.

McCormack, B., Kitson, A., Harvey, G., Rycroft-Malone, J., Titchen, A., & Seers, K. (2002). Getting evidence into practice: The meaning of 'context.' *Journal of Advanced Nursing, 38*(1), 94-104.

Meredith, S., Feldman, P. H., Frey, D., Giammarco, L., Hall, K., Arnold, K., Brown, N. J., & Ray, W. A. (2002). Improving medication use in home healthcare patients: A randomized controlled trial. *Journal of the American Geriatrics Society, 50,* 1484-1491.

Meredith, S., Feldman, P. H., Frey, D., Hall, K., Arnold, K., Brown, N. J., & Ray, W. A. (2001). Possible medication errors in home healthcare patients. *Journal of the American Geriatrics Society, 49,* 719-724.

Monane, M., Matthias, D. M., Nagle, B. A., & Kelly, M. A. (1998). Improving prescribing patterns for the elderly through an online drug utilization review intervention: A system linking the physician, pharmacist, and computer. *Journal of the American Medical Association, 280*(14), 1249-1252.

Murphy, A., & McDonald, J. (2004). Power, status and marginalisation: Rural social workers and evidence-based practice in multidisciplinary teams. *Australian Social Work, 57*(2), 127-136.

National Center for Health Statistics. (2004). Health, United States, 2004. Atlanta, GA: Center for Disease Control and Prevention.

National Center for HIV Prevention. (2003). Procedural Guidance for Selected Strategies and Interventions for Community-Based Organizations Funded Under Program Announcement. Atlanta, GA: Centers for Disease Control and Prevention.

Phillips, D. P., Christenfeld, N., & Glynn, L. M. (1998). Increase in US medication-error deaths between 1983 and 1993. *The Lancet, 351*(9103), 643-644.

Quality Interagency Coordination Task Force. (2000). Doing What Counts for Patient Safety: Federal Actions to Reduce Medical Errors and Their Impact. Rockville, MD: Agency for Healthcare Research and Quality.

Rogers, E. (1995). Diffusion of innovations (4th ed.). New York: Free Press.

Rossi, P. H., Lipsey, M. W., & Freeman, H. E. (2004). Evaluation: A systematic approach (7th ed.). Thousand Oaks, CA: Sage Publications.

Rycroft-Malone, J., Harvey, G., Seers, K., Kitson, A., McCormack, B., & Titchen, A. (2004). An exploration of the factors that influence the implementation of evidence into practice. *Journal of Clinical Nursing, 13*(8), 913-924.

Rycroft-Malone, J., Kitson, A., Harvey, G., McCormack, B., Seers, K., Titchen, A., & Estabrooks, C. (2002). Ingredients for change: Revisiting a conceptual framework. *Quality & Safety in Health Care, 11*(2), 174-180.

Rycroft-Malone, J., Seers, K., Titchen, A., Harvey, G., Kitson, A., & McCormack, B. (2004). What counts as evidence in evidence-based practice? *Journal of Advanced Nursing, 47*(1), 81-90.

Silverman, J. B., Stapinski, C. D., Huber, C., Ghandi, T. K., & Churchill, W. W. (2004). Computer-based system for preventing adverse drug events. *American Journal of Health System Pharmacy, 61*(15), 1599-1603.

Tamblyn, R., Huang, A., Perreault, R., Jacques, A., Roy, D., Hanley, J., McLeod, P., & Laprise, R. (2003). The medical office of the 21st century: Effectiveness of computerized decision-making support in reducing inappropriate prescribing in primary care. *Canadian Medical Association Journal, 169*(6), 549-556.

The Commonwealth Fund. (2004). The Commonwealth Fund Health Care Opinion Leaders Survey. New York.

Titler, M. G. (2004). Methods in translation science. *Worldviews Evidence-Based Nursing, 1*(1), 38-48.

Walshe, K., & Rundall, T. (2001). Evidence-based management: From theory to practice in health care. *Milbank Quarterly, 79*(3), 429-457.

Weiss, C. H. (1997). Evaluation (2nd ed.). New York: Prentice Hall.

Weissert, W., Chernew, M., & Hirth, R. (2003). Titrating versus targeting home care services to frail elderly clients: An application of agency theory and cost-benefit analysis to home care policy. *Journal of Aging and Health, 15*(1), 99-123.

Wholey, J. S., Hatry, H. P., & Newcomer, K. E. (Eds.). (2004). Handbook of practical program evaluation (2nd ed.). New York: Jossey-Bass.

Wu, S.-Y., & Green, A. (2000). Projection of chronic illness and cost inflation. Santa Monica, CA: Rand Corporation.

Zhan, C., Sangl, J., Bierman, A. S., Miller, M. R., Friedman, B., Wickizer, S. W., & Meyer, G. S. (2001). Potentially inappropriate medication use in the community-dwelling elderly: Findings from the 1996 Medical Expenditure Panel Survey. *Journal of the American Medical Association, 286*(22), 2823-2829.

Evidence-Based Interventions
in Fall Prevention

Jon Pynoos, PhD
Debra Rose, PhD
Laurence Rubenstein, MD, MPH
In Hee Choi, MIPA
Dory Sabata, OTD, OTR/L

SUMMARY. Falls and fall-related injuries, prevalent among older
adults, not only have devastating consequences for older adults in
terms of morbidity and mortality, but are also associated with high
health care costs. Studies have found that multifactorial intervention
strategies can effectively prevent and/or reduce falls among older
adults. The purpose of this article is to describe evidence-based intervention strategies for community-dwelling older adults. Fall prevention efforts are clearly an important area of health promotion and injury
prevention, and evidence presented in this article provides support for

Jon Pynoos is Co-Director, Fall Prevention Center of Excellence and UPS Foundation, Professor of Gerontology, Policy, Planning and Development, Andrus Gerontology Center, University of Southern California. Debra Rose is Co-Director, Fall
Prevention Center of Excellence and Co-Director, Center for Successful Aging, California State University, Fullerton. Laurence Rubenstein is Co-Director, Fall Prevention Center of Excellence and Director, Geriatric Research Education and Clinical
Center, VA Greater Los Angeles Healthcare System. In Hee Choi is a Doctoral Stu-
dent, University of Southern California School of Gerontology and Research Assistant,
Fall Prevention Center of Excellence. Dory Sabata is Occupational Therapist and Research Associate, Fall Prevention Center of Excellence.

[Haworth co-indexing entry note]: "Evidence-Based Interventions in Fall Prevention." Pynoos, Jon et al.
Co-published simultaneously in *Home Health Care Services Quarterly* (The Haworth Press, Inc.) Vol. 25,
No. 1/2, 2006, pp. 55-73; and: *Evidence-Based Interventions for Community Dwelling Older Adults* (ed: Su-
san M. Enguídanos) The Haworth Press, Inc., 2006, pp. 55-73. Single or multiple copies of this article are
available for a fee from The Haworth Document Delivery Service [1-800-HAWORTH, 9:00 a.m. - 5:00 p.m.
(EST). E-mail address: docdelivery@haworthpress.com].

effective intervention strategies. Home health care professionals can play a significant role in such intervention strategies. However, further research is needed to clarify which groups will benefit most from specific intervention programs. *[Article copies available for a fee from The Haworth Document Delivery Service: 1-800-HAWORTH. E-mail address: <docdelivery@haworthpress.com> Website: <http://www.HaworthPress.com> © 2006 by The Haworth Press, Inc. All rights reserved.]*

KEYWORDS. Community-based programs, community-dwelling older adults, environmental modification, fall, home health care professional, physical activity, multifactorial intervention strategies, risk assessment

INTRODUCTION

Falls and fall-related injuries are prevalent among older adults. Studies have reported that 30% to 60% of community-dwelling older adults fall each year, and the fall incidence rates for this population range from 0.2 to 1.6 falls per person per year, with a mean of approximately 0.7 falls per year (Rubenstein, Castle, Diener, Hooker, Jones, & Vasquez, 2004). Falls not only have devastating consequences for older adults in terms of morbidity and mortality, but are also associated with high acute and long-term care costs. In 1994, total direct cost of fall injuries among people 65 and older was $20.2 billion (Centers for Disease Control and Prevention, 2004). Stevens (2004) also reported that the total cost of all fall injuries for people age 65 or older is expected to reach $43.8 billion by 2020 (in current dollars). However, falls and fall-related injuries are potentially preventable public health problems. A number of studies have found that multifactorial intervention programs can effectively prevent and/or reduce a substantial proportion of falls among older adults (Gillespie et al., 2004; RAND, 2003), thereby improving their independent functioning and enhancing their quality of life.

The purpose of this article is to describe evidence-based intervention strategies that have been effective in reducing fall incidence rates and fall-related injuries among community-dwelling older adults. First, it provides a brief overview of fall incidence among older adults in terms of frequency and location, as well as risk factors associated with falls. Second, the article examines the content and effectiveness of recent evidence-based intervention programs designed to prevent falls. Third, it discusses challenges related to evidence-based intervention practice in fall prevention, as well as the role of home health care professionals in this field.

BACKGROUND

Where and How People Fall

Falls and fall-related injuries, a potentially preventable public health problem, have been the leading cause of injury deaths among older adults (Stevens, 2002/2003). In 2001, approximately 1.6 million elders were treated in hospital emergency departments, and 373,000 were hospitalized for fall-related injuries (Stevens, 2002/2003). In addition, more than 11,600 people aged 65 and older died from fall-related injuries (CDC, 2004). Fall-related hip fractures account for approximately 25 percent of injury deaths among those over age 65, and 34 percent of injury deaths among those aged 85 or older (Peek-Asa & Zwerling, 2003).

Data compiled from the 1997 and 1998 National Health Interview Survey indicate that the majority (55%) of fall injuries among older people occurred inside the house (Kochera, 2002). Josephson and colleagues (1991) also reported that the home environment is implicated in 35%-40% of falls among older persons. An additional 23% of falls occurred outside but near the house and 22% occurred away from the home (Kochera, 2002). Older adults become less mobile and spend more of their day inside their dwelling units, which may account for the greater number of injuries in the home.

Given the increasing number of older adults with functional limitations who are at risk of falling, the negative consequences of falls and the associated health care costs, significant efforts have been made to develop and test fall prevention interventions. Researchers have investigated the efficacy of fall prevention intervention strategies designed to reduce the risk factors associated with falls, as well as the actual incidence of falls and fall-related injuries among older adults.

Risk Factors Associated with Falls

Risk factors associated with falls include intrinsic factors (e.g., age-related physiological changes, impairments to the sensory-nervous system, disorders of the musculoskeletal system, and specific acute and chronic diseases) as well as extrinsic factors (e.g., environmental hazards and obstacles interfering with safe mobility, and medication side effects) (Steinberg, Cartwright, Peel, & Williams, 2000; Tideiksaar, 2001).

In general, intrinsic risk factors include chronic diseases, muscle weaknesses, gait disorders, and mental status alterations, all of which can have additive effects. Rawsky investigated 100 articles published from 1979 to 1996 which were related to falls among the elderly population in a variety of settings, and identified the following as the most often cited intrinsic risk factors: cognitive impairment/psychological status, acute/chronic illness and mobility problems, sensory deficits, and fall history (Perrell, Nelson, Goldman, Luther, Prieto-Lewis, & Rubenstein, 2001). Many age-related changes, including declines in sensory and integrative systems in older adults, increase the risk of falls. For example, studies have found that (1) weakness in the lower extremities is the most potent risk factor associated with falls, increasing the odds of falling, on average, by more than four times; and (2) gait and balance impairments are significant risk factors for falls, associated with about a three-fold increase in the risk of falling (Rubenstein & Josephson, 2002/2003).

Some of the most common extrinsic factors affecting the risk of falling include: (1) poor or inadequate lighting, (2) changes in floor surface or slippery surfaces (e.g., wet floors and non-slip-resistant bathtub surfaces), (3) high-gloss floors and/or walking surfaces, (4) problems associated with stairs (e.g., stairways without handrail support), (5) inappropriate chair or cabinet heights, (6) clutter, storage problems, and tripping hazards such as furniture or throw rugs, and (7) poor sidewalk and pavement conditions (Dickinson, Shroyer, Elias, Curry, & Cook, 2004; Leslie & Pierre, 1999; Norton, Campbell, Lee-Joe, Robinson, & Butler, 1997; Tideiksaar, 2001). Extrinsic factors (e.g., environmental hazards or hazardous activities, medication side effects) generally create conditions that lead to trips or slips, and thereby pose a greater risk for community-dwelling older adults who may already have multiple intrinsic risk factors for falls in particular (Perrell, Nelson, Goldman, Luther, Prieto-Lewis, & Rubenstein, 2001). Moreover, the relationship between medication use and falls has been investigated in many studies, which have found that: (1) the use of psychotropic medications, antidepressants, anti-arrhythmic heart medications, and digoxin significantly increases the risk of falls; and (2) the use of three or more medications is clinically and statistically related to the risk of falls (Cumming, 1998; Leipzig, Cumming, & Tinetti, 1999; Rubenstein & Josephson, 2002/2003).

The majority of falls result from a complex interaction between such intrinsic and extrinsic factors, and in general, the relationship between falls and environmental factors is complex and individual specific (Leslie & Pierre, 1999).

The Need for Evidence-Based Practice

Evidence-based practice refers to intervention strategies supported by rigorous, systematic, and objective research. According to Altpeter and colleagues (2006), using an evidence-based health promotion approach has many advantages in terms of increasing the likelihood of successful outcomes, and enhancing the ability to identify common health indicators and match health programs to those risks and conditions. This approach is beneficial to programs for both increasing effective use of resources and validating or expanding an existing program. Evidence-based fall prevention research can be translated into practice and used to design the most effective interventions based on the needs and characteristics of a given population, and to help implement cost-effective intervention fall prevention programs.

OVERVIEW OF RESEARCH FINDINGS

Various types of intervention strategies aimed at fall prevention have been implemented with different target populations (e.g., healthy and frail community-residing older adults, nursing-home residents) and in a variety of settings (e.g., homes, communities, long-term-care facilities, hospitals) (Rose, 2002/2003). In general, these intervention strategies include, but are not limited to: (1) fall risk assessment and management (including medication management), (2) physical activity-based interventions, (3) environmental modifications, (4) education, (5) assistive devices, (6) visual interventions, and (7) footwear interventions. This article focuses on four major intervention strategies (fall risk assessment and management, physical activity, environmental modifications, and education) along with multifactorial intervention strategies, which have been proven to be the most effective in reducing fall incidence rates and fall-related injuries among older adults at high risk for falls.

Major Intervention Strategies

Stand-alone Intervention Programs

Stand-alone intervention programs (e.g., environmental modifications, staff education, or fall prevention education for older adults) are frequently used with the intent of reducing falls. However, they have generally been less effective than multi-factorial interventions. (American Geriatrics Society, British Geriatrics Society, and American Academy of Orthopedic Surgeons Panel on Fall Prevention, 2001; Gillespie et al., 2000; Peek-Asa & Zwerling, 2003; Roberts, 2003; Tinetti, 2003). A meta-analysis conducted by the RAND Corporation compared the effectiveness of different types of fall prevention interventions. Of the four types of interventions (fall risk assessment and management; physical activity; environmental modification; and education), the RAND study determined that a fall risk assessment with a follow-up management program was the most effective single intervention with physical activity ranking second as a stand alone program.

1. Fall Risk Assessment and Management Programs

Since falls result from a complex interaction between intrinsic and extrinsic risk factors, identifying the predisposing and precipitating factors related to falls is critical. In general, the major components of a fall risk assessment and management program include (1) a questionnaire to identify risk factors for falls, which can be self-administered or used by a professional; (2) medical evaluation (e.g., gait, balance, strength, vision, postural vital signs, medication review, cognitive and functional status); and (3) follow-up interventions such as a tailored physical activity program, environmental modifications, medical risk factor reduction, and assistive devices (Chang et al., 2004; RAND, 2003).

According to Perrell and colleagues (2001), three types of assessments relevant to falls and mobility have been conducted on the basis of setting- or discipline-specific factors: (1) comprehensive medical assessments performed by geriatricians or nurse practitioners in outpatient or nursing home settings, (2) nursing fall risk assessments completed in hospital and nursing home settings, and (3) functional mobility assessments completed by physical therapists or physicians in an outpatient setting.

Studies have found that risk assessment and management has been an effective means of preventing falls. For example, a study by Close et al. (1999) found that a medical assessment at a day hospital after discharge–followed by an occupational therapy assessment at home, with direct intervention advice, education, and referral–resulted in a reduction in the number of falls over one year. Tinetti (2003) also reported that multifactorial assessments followed by interventions targeting the identified risk factors (e.g., a combination of review and possible reduction of medications; balance and gait training, muscle-strengthening physical activity; evaluation of postural blood pressure, followed by strategies to reduce any decreases in postural blood pressure; home hazard modifications; together with targeted medical and cardiovascular assessments and treatments) have been shown to reduce the occurrence of falling by 25 to 39 percent.

2. Physical Activity

As older adults are more likely to experience declines in physical functioning with advancing age, physical activity interventions designed to reduce or reverse these declines can be effective in preventing falls. Physical activity interventions range from single exercise forms (e.g., resistance exercises, walking, cycling, tai chi) to multi component exercise programs (e.g., aerobic endurance, flexibility, strength, and balance training) (Rose, 2002/2003). In general, physical activity programs tailored to enhance gait and balance, combined with muscle strengthening and flexibility, have proven to be effective in fall prevention. Even though some physical activity-only interventions have not been judged as effective, depending on the level of fall risk studied, interventions that included balance training as a major element significantly reduced the occurrence of falls among older adults (Province et al., 1995).

Numerous studies have reported the benefits of physical activity, either as a stand-alone intervention strategy or as a major component of a multifactorial intervention strategy, in reducing fall risk and fall incidence rates in the older adult population (Rose, 2004). Traditional forms of exercise, as well as tai chi, an eastern form of physical activity which consists of a comprehensive series of gentle physical movements and breathing techniques, have proven to be effective stand-alone physical activity interventions for relatively healthy but sedentary community-residing older adults as well as adults at moderate risk for falls. Wolf et al. (1996) reported that a 15-week tai chi intervention program among persons aged 70 and older living in the community reduced the risk of multiple falls by 47.5%, indicating that a tai chi intervention can impact favorably on the occurrence of falls in a group of older adults at moderate risk for falls. More recently, Li and colleagues (2005) have demonstrated significant improvements in multiple measures of balance, physical performance, and fear-of-falling in a group of sedentary older adults participating in a six-month program. The intervention group also experienced significantly fewer falls of any kind as well as injurious falls during the six-month follow-up period, compared to a group who received a low intensity flexibility intervention. As effective as this form of physical activity appears to be for low-to-moderate risk groups, it appears to be less effective as a stand-alone fall prevention strategy in groups of older adults who are more frail or transitioning into frailty (Wolf et al., 2003).

According to the RAND meta-analyses (2003), physical activity interventions, which typically included cardiovascular endurance, muscular strength, flexibility, and/or balance, reduced the risk of falls by 12% and the number of falls by 19%. The multi centered *Frailty and Injuries: Co-operative Studies on Intervention Techniques (FICSIT)* randomized, controlled trials also showed that physical activity intervention programs conducted in five community-settings and 2 nursing home settings significantly reduced the risk of falls among older adults (Province et al., 1995). Although each study included a physical activity component, the interventions varied with respect to the type of physical activity used and the intensity, frequency, and duration of the intervention. Specifically, the combined multi site outcomes demonstrated a significant reduction in the risk of falling for the interventions that included a non-tailored physical activity component (13% reduction) and a 24% reduction in fall risk if the intervention included specific balance and gait activities. In general, group-based or individualized physical activity interventions that are characterized by higher levels of intensity, frequency, and duration are associated with greater reduction in fall risk (Berg & Kairy, 2002/2003). Moreover, individuals who demonstrate higher levels of compliance during a physical activity intervention also achieve better functional outcomes as indicated by Shumway-Cook et al. (1997) in a study that combined a twice-weekly intensive out-patient program (two days per week) with a home program that included muscle strengthening, flexibility, and balance. The more compliant intervention subjects demonstrated a 33% reduction in falls while their less compliant subjects demonstrated only an 11% reduction in fall risk (Shumway-Cook, Gruber, Baldwin, & Liao, 1997).

Despite the positive outcomes that have been shown in many published studies, the optimal type of physical activity, as well as frequency, intensity and duration of the activity-based falls prevention intervention requires further investigation. Rose (2002/2003) recommends that future research should: (1) identify the minimum dosage (i.e., frequency, intensity, and duration) of physical activity needed to significantly lower fall incidence rates and fall-related injuries among older adults at different levels of risk; (2) compare the relative benefits of different types of physical activity interventions; (3) investigate the cost effectiveness and cost savings associated with different types of intervention strategies; (4) identify which type of intervention strategy is most effective for older adults with cognitive impairment and dementia; and (5) address how the effectiveness of a given physical activity intervention is influenced by the ethnicity of the participants.

Not only is the type of physical activity an important consideration, but also the setting. To date, group-based physical activity interventions have been most often studied. However, a few studies that have investigated individualized physical activity programs in the home have also demonstrated significant outcomes. For example, Campbell et al. (1997; 1999) demonstrated a significant reduction in the rate of falling in a group of older women (80 years and older) who participated in a moderate intensity home-based program three times per week for six months. Participants received an individualized program designed and initially instructed by a physical therapist but then continued to exercise without supervision for the remainder of the intervention period. They were also encouraged to walk an additional three times per week. Motivation to remain in the study was enhanced through regular telephone follow-up. Particularly noteworthy was the fact that those participants who continued with the program for an additional year after the end of the study (71% of original group) also experience reduced fall rates during the second year when compared to the non-exercising control group. It has also been shown that home-bound frail elderly also benefit from physical activity interventions that target balance and gait, strength, and flexibility.

3. Environmental Modifications

In general, the homes and communities of older persons often have numerous hazards, dangerous areas and a lack of supportive features, all of which can contribute to falls (Pynoos, Sabata, Abernethy, Alley, Nishita, & Overton, 2004). For example, Gill et al. (2000) found that the prevalence of environmental hazards was high in most homes; nearly all homes had at least two potential hazards. The purpose of environmental modification strategies is, therefore, to reduce and/or eliminate extrinsic risk factors associated with falls. Given that the majority of older adults prefer to remain in their homes and communities, environmental modification interventions are particularly important.

Environmental modifications, particularly home modifications, attempt to reestablish an equilibrium between a person whose capabilities have declined and the demands of the environment (Lawton & Nahemow, 1973). Such interventions include not only abating hazards but also adding supportive features (e.g., grab bars, handrails, ramps). To date, however, the majority of studies investigating the association between environmental modifications and fall prevention have focused on hazard abatement/reduction.

Studies have yielded mixed results as to the role of environmental modifications in fall prevention. For example, Gill, Williams, and Tinetti (2000) reported that the association between environmental hazards and nonsyncopal falls was not firmly established. Kochera (2002) also reported that studies have been unclear about whether a comprehensive program of home modifications leads directly to a reduction in the incidence and severity of falls, although researchers generally agree that home modifications are an important way to promote safety and independent living. Home modifications interventions have demonstrated success when a more skilled professional (e.g., occupational therapist) conducts a home assessment and assists with the home modification process as indicated by a study by Cumming et al. (1999): the authors found that 36% of the subjects in the intervention group had at least one fall during follow-up, compared with 45% of the controls (p = .05) (Cumming et al., 1999). There is also evidence that home modifications may be more effective at reducing falls among those with a prior history of falls (Salkeld, Cumming, O'Neil, Thomas, Szony, & Westbury, 2000). Accordingly, the overall consensus from RAND's meta-analysis (2003) and other studies (CDC, 2004; Roberts, 2003) is that the best approach is to include home modification in a multifactorial strategy for fall prevention.

Yet to be determined, however, is the extent to which environmental problems contribute to fall incidence rates and fall-related injuries, as well as the types of environmental modification interventions most likely to have an impact (Pynoos, Sabata, & Choi, 2004). The availability of trained personnel to conduct the initial home assessment and adequate funding to hire qualified individuals to complete the modifications are also important considerations in the success of any environmental modification strategy (Pynoos, Sabata, Abernethy, Alley, Nishita, & Overton, 2004).

4. Education

Raising awareness of the potential consequences of falling and enhancing knowledge about fall prevention strategies are the major goals of educational interventions. To date, studies have shown that education as a sole intervention is ineffective (Tinetti, 2003). However, multifactorial interventions that have included behavioral and educational programs have demonstrated benefits in terms of reducing falls (American Geriatrics Society, British Geriatrics Society, and American Academy of Orthopedic Surgeons Panel on Fall prevention, 2001).

Another approach to education is to raise awareness among health care and community service providers. Providers who become more aware of the issue of fall prevention can work together to provide more comprehensive care. For example, the Connecticut Collaboration for Fall Prevention (CCFP) developed educational materials for physicians, care planners, and home health providers to screen for risk factors and become aware of available services to aid in preventing falls. This systems approach to managing fall risk within a community resulted in increased intervention and referral when risk factors such as gait and balance problems were identified (Fortinsky et al., 2004).

Multifactorial Intervention Programs

Although single interventions may be more practical to implement, RAND researchers (2003) suggest that the most potent interventions are multi-component interventions that combine an initial risk assessment with physical activity, education and/or environmental inspection/modification strategies. In particular, it is recommended that multifactorial interventions for community-dwelling older persons should include: gait and balance training, advice on the appropriate use of assistive devices, review and modification of medications with special attention to psychotropic drugs. Additionally, treatment of postural hypotension, modification of environmental hazards, and treatment of cardiovascular disorders, including cardiac arrhythmias are effective components of fall prevention interventions (Rubenstein, Castle, Diener, Hooker, Jones, & Vasquez, 2004).

A number of multifactorial interventions have proven effective in fall prevention. For example, Yates and Dunnagan (2001) investigated a multifactorial approach with a 10-week program of home based physical activity, nutritional counseling and/or referral, and environmental hazard education. The 10-week physical activity program in this intervention focused on improving strength, coordination, balance, and mobility through 19 chair-based activities. Nutritional education and screening were based on the Nutritional Screening Initiative. Environmental risks within the bathroom, kitchen, living room, bedroom, stairwells, and yard were identified using a 40-question environmental in-home assessment. Yates and Dunnagan (2001) concluded that the intervention group showed statistically significant improvement in balance, bicep endurance, lower extremity power, reduction of environmental hazards, falls efficacy, and nutritious food behavior during the study period.

Day et al. (2002) examined the effectiveness of three interventions among a group of relatively healthy community-dwelling older adults: group based physical activity, home hazard management, and vision improvement in fall prevention, alone and in combination. Participants received a home visit by a trained assessor. Participants in the intervention group attended a weekly one-hour physical activity class for 15 weeks, supplemented with a daily home physical activity program designed to improve flexibility, leg strength, and balance. With respect to home hazard management, participants in the intervention group removed or modified home hazards either by themselves or via the City of Whitehorse's home maintenance program through which home maintenance staff visited the home and provided a quote for the work, including free labor and materials to the value of $100. In addition, each participant was referred to his/her eye care provider, general practitioner, or local optometrist if his/her vision tested below predetermined criteria. Results indicated that the group-based physical activity component was the most potent single intervention tested, with an estimated reduction in fall incidence rates of 6.9% over the 18-month study period. A combination of all three strategies, however, resulted in a further reduction in estimated fall incidence rates (14%) (Day et al., 2002).

Similarly, findings from a study by Tinetti et al. (1994) demonstrated that multifactorial intervention programs had a positive impact on falls reduction with the intervention group demonstrating a significantly lower incidence of falls during the post-intervention follow-up period. This study investigated a strategy of mixed interventions (physical training, education, and behavioral recommendations, environmental interventions and home modifications) in a group of 301 community-dwelling individuals age 70 years or older. Participants in the intervention group received a combination of adjustment in their medications, behavioral instructions, and physical activity programs aimed at modifying their risk factors. Tinetti et al. (1994) found that 35 percent of the intervention group fell, as compared to 47 percent of the control group (p = 0.04) during one year of follow-up. Consequently, Tinetti et al. (1994) concluded that a multiple-risk-factor intervention strategy resulted in a significant reduction in the risk of falling among elderly persons in the community.

In general, a multifactorial intervention strategy enhances the power of an intervention, but at the same time, it is more time and resource-intensive and requires a multidisciplinary team of providers that can include emergency room physicians and nurses, general practitioners, physical and occupational therapists, pharmacists, psychiatrists, and social workers (Rose, 2002/2003). A stable funding source for sustaining and expanding existing programs and services to older adults, and for securing qualified personnel and/or training personnel to implement these intervention programs, is also crucial. However, to date, few studies have examined what components of the intervention have the strongest effects, in what combination, and the interplay between multiple risk reduction strategies.

Another important issue is the compliance of older adults with the designs and implementation of intervention programs. In order to make such intervention programs effective, older adults must be willing to make the necessary changes to their lifestyles and home environments. To do so, the goals of an intervention program should be compatible, easy to implement, and affordable.

State Initiated/Community-Based Fall Prevention Program

In the state of California, several demonstration programs have begun to address the issue of fall prevention at a local level. Many of these programs are offered in group settings and within local communities, and one example is the No More Falls demonstration project that utilizes an initial risk assessment and follow-up plan. Participants in the No More Falls program are at least 65 years old and live in the community. The intervention consists of: (1) a comprehensive health assessment modified to include fall risk identification; (2) an individualized fall prevention action plan listing activities to reduce identified fall risk factors; (3) individual counseling and education about care plan goals and activities; and (4) either a home hazard assessment checklist for client self-appraisal and/or the offer to have program staff conduct a home visit to evaluate, assess and abate hazards to intervention groups (Rose et al., 2004). The results of the initial pilot study have been promising in that program participants were 20% less likely to fall one year after completing the program (Rose et al., 2004).

The FallProof™ program is an example of a targeted physical activity program that is group based and currently operating in multiple community-based centers in Southern California. Specialized training is required to become an instructor of the program. Physical activity instructors with previous experience working with older adults are trained to conduct a comprehensive risk assessment to determine program eligibility and also select the appropriate types of balance and mobility activities for the identified impairments. The FallProof™ program is designed to be implemented in a group setting such as a senior center or community recreation center. Initially, the program was tested in 18 senior centers in Orange County. Evidence of reduced fall risk was demonstrated after only 16 training sessions, as well as improved functional performance and greater balance-related self-confidence (Rose, 2002).

The Community and Home Injury Prevention Program for Seniors (CHIPPS) also utilizes a community-based approach to fall prevention. This health promotion program is designed to prevent injuries among seniors, and currently operates in San Francisco. It educates home care workers, caregivers, and medical providers about fall prevention and other injuries of older adults. The program provides home safety assessments and minor home modifications such as grab bars to low income seniors. One study of the program found that it was able to reduce fall incidence by almost 60% among relatively healthy seniors.

Low-to-Moderate Risk vs. High Risk Populations

Community-dwelling elderly are a heterogeneous group when it comes to being at risk for falling. According to the American Geriatrics Society (2001), high-risk older adults are those individuals with recurrent falls, those living in a nursing home, persons prone to injurious falls, or persons presenting after a fall. Given the differences between low-to-moderate risk populations and high risk populations, effective intervention programs have tailored their interventions to the specific needs of the target population.

With respect to fall risk assessment and management processes, the degree of intensity for an assessment varies by target population. For example, older adults in a relatively low-risk population can have fall risk screening assessments conducted as part of routine primary healthcare visits, whereas older people in high-risk groups may require a more comprehensive and detailed assessment to fully elucidate the complex nature of the risk and to plan therapy (Rubenstein et al., 2002/2003). In terms of physical activity interventions, multi-component physical activity programs are generally more effective for reducing fall risks in community-residing older adults at low-to-moderate risk for falls, whereas individualized physical activity interventions targeting specific physical impairments are likely to be more effective in reducing fall rates and fall-related injuries among those at high risk for falls or with a history of falls (Rose, 2002/2003).

Implications for Practice: The Role of Home Health Care Professionals

Home health care professionals can play a pivotal role in assessing and managing fall risks in home and community-based settings. Home health providers who see older adults regularly may be the first to recognize the need for a geriatric risk assessment. Some home health professionals such as nurses, physical therapists and occupational therapists may be involved in conducting parts of the fall risk assessment or environmental assessments. Physical activity programs may be taught by home health providers for use as a home program or referrals may be made to community-based group physical activity programs. As home health care providers are most likely to have regular contacts with older adults, they are in an excellent position to encourage their clients to continue their involvement with programs such as exercise and to make their homes safer and more supportive. Home health providers may also make recommendations for home modifications and assistive devices to encourage physical activity and safe participation in everyday activities. Aside from providing interventions to a single individual, home health providers also can participate in a larger system or network of service providers promoting fall prevention.

CONCLUSION

In the past decade, there has been a dramatic increase in fall prevention research. Studies have found that various intervention programs can effectively prevent falls. In particular, multifactorial intervention programs that target both intrinsic and extrinsic risk factors have been shown to be the most effective in reducing falls among older adults, thereby improving their independent functioning and enhancing their quality of life. Furthermore, multidisciplinary team efforts, which include cooperation among public health professionals, community-based organizations, and government agencies, are vital for successful fall prevention.

Fall prevention efforts are an important area of health promotion and injury prevention. Many falls are preventable, and evidence presented in this article provides support for effective intervention strategies, even though further research is needed to clarify which groups may benefit the most from specific intervention programs. Providers of home and community-based services can carry out assessments and interventions that target fall risk reduction. By utilizing measures of fall risk factors with demonstrated reliability and validity, providers can better understand the underlying issues that put a person at risk of falls. When providers are familiar with research and recognize the evidence that supports a particular intervention or service, then effective programs and services can be developed. Research can be translated into practice when programs that have demonstrated effectiveness are replicated in a similar manner in the practice setting.

Groups around the country are trying to build on what we know works to reduce falls by raising awareness of fall prevention and intervention strategies. A National Fall Prevention Summit was held recently to develop a national action plan for fall prevention (The National Council on the Aging, 2005). Within the state of California, the Archstone Foundation is supporting a statewide Fall Prevention Initiative. The Fall Prevention Center of Excellence, the driving force of the California initiative, will provide training and technical assistance to providers, as well as help identify and develop model programs in fall prevention (www.stopfalls. org). The work of the Connecticut Collaboration for Fall Prevention (CCFP) also demonstrates that with training and education, providers can better identify those at risk for falls and offer needed services. Each of these efforts requires the skills and contributions of home health providers who interact with older adults in their homes and communities.

REFERENCES

Altpeter, M., Bryant, L., Schneider, E., & Whitelaw, N. (2006). Evidence-based health promotion: Knowing and using what works for older adults. *Home Health Care Services Quarterly*, 25(1/2), 1-11.

American Geriatrics Society, British Geriatrics Society, and American Academy of Orthopedic Surgeons Panel on Fall prevention. (2001). Guideline for the prevention of falls in older persons. *Journal of American Geriatrics Society*, 49(5), 664-672.

Berg, K.O., & Kairy, D. (2002/2003). Balance interventions to prevent falls. *Generations*, 26(4), 75-78.

Campbell, A.J., Robertson, M.C., Gardner, M.M., Norton, R.N., & Buchner, D.M. (1999). Falls prevention over 2 years: A randomized controlled trial in women 80 years and older. *Age and Ageing*, 28, 513-518.

Campbell, A.J., Robertson, M.C., Gardner, M.M., Norton, R.N., Tilyard, M.W., & Buchner, D.M. (1997). Randomised controlled trial of a general practice programme of home based exercise to prevent falls in elderly women. *British Medical Journal*, 315(7115), 1065-1069.

Centers for Disease Control and Prevention (CDC). (2004). Falls and hip fractures among older adults. Retrieved September 15, 2004, from *http://www.cdc.gov/ncipc/factsheets/falls.htm*.

Chang, J.T., Morton, S.C., Rubenstein, L.Z., Mojica, W.A., Maglione, M., Suttorp, M.J., Roth, E.A., & Shekelle, P.G. (2004). Interventions for the prevention of falls in older adults: Systematic review and meta-analysis of randomized clinical trials. *British Medical Journal*, 328(7441), 680-688.

Close, J., Ellis, M., Hooper, R., Glucksman, E., Jackson, S., & Swift, C. (1999) Prevention of falls in the elderly trial (PROFET): A randomized controlled trial. *Lancet*, *353*, 93-97.

Cumming, R.G. (1998). Epidemiology of medication-related falls and fractures in the elderly. *Drugs and Aging*, 12(2), 43-53.

Cumming, R.G., Thomas, M., Szonyi, G., Salkeld, G., O'Neill, E., Westbury, C., & Frampton, G. (1999). Home visits by an occupational therapist for assessment and modification of environmental hazards: A randomized trial of fall prevention. *Journal of the American Geriatric Society*, *47*, 1397-1402.

Day, L., Fildes, B., Gordon, I., Fitzharris, M., Flamer, H., & Lord, S. (2002). Randomised factorial trial of fall prevention among older people living in their own homes. *British Medical Journal*, 325, 128-131.

Dickinson, J.I., Shroyer, J.L., Elia, J.W., Curry, Z.D., & Cook, C.E. (2004). Preventing falls with interior design. *Journal of Family and Consumer Sciences*, 96(2), 13-20.

Fall Prevention Center of Excellence website. (2005). http://www.stopfalls.org/

Fortinsky, R. H., Iannuzzi-Suchch, M., Baker, D. I., Gottschalk, M., King, M. B., Brown, C. J., & Tinetti, M. E. (2004). Fall-risk assessment and management in clinical practice: Views from health care providers. *Journal of the American Geriatric Society*, 52, 1522-1526.

Gill, T.M., Williams, C.S., & Tinetti, M.E. (2000). Environmental hazards and the risk of nonsyncopal falls in the homes of community-living older persons. *Medical Care*, 38(12), 1174-1183.

Gillespie, L.D., Gillespie, W.J., Robertson, M.C. et al. (2004). Interventions for preventing falls in elderly people (Cochrane Review). In The Cochrane Library, issue 3. Oxford, United Kingdom: Update Software Ltd., 2004.

Josephson, K., Febacher, D., & Rubenstein, L.Z. (1991). Home safety and fall prevention. *Clinical Geriatric Medicine*, *7*, 707-731.

Kochera, A. (2002). Falls among older persons and the role of the home: An analysis of cost, incidence, and potential savings from home modification. Issue Brief. *Public Policy Institute American Association of Retired Persons*, IB56, 1-14. Retrieved September 15, 2004, from *http://research.aarp.org/il/ib56_falls.html*.

Lawton, M.P. & Nahemow, L. (1973). Ecology and the aging process. In C. Eisdorfer and M.P. Lawton (Eds.), *Psychology of adult development and aging*. Washington D. C.: American Psychological Association.

Leipzig, R.M., Cumming, R.G., & Tinetti, M.E. (1999). Drugs and falls in older people: A systematic review and meta-analysis: I. Psychotropic drugs. *Journal of the American Geriatrics Society*, *47*(1), 30-39.

Leslie, M., & Pierre, R.W. (1999). An integrated risk assessment approach to fall prevention among community-dwelling elderly. *American Journal of Health Studies*, 15(2), 57-62.

Li, F., Harmer, P., Fisher, K.J., McAuley, E., Chaumeton, N., Eckstrom, E., & Wilson, N.E. (2005). Tai chi and fall reductions in older adults: A randomized controlled trial. *Journal of Gerontology: Biological Sciences and Medical Sciences*, 60A(2), 187-194.

Norton, R., Campbell, A.J., Lee-Joe, T., Robinson, E., & Butler, M. (1997). Circumstances of falls resulting in hip fractures among older people. *Journal of the American Geriatrics Society*, 45(9), 1108-1112.

Peek-Asa, C., & Zwerling, C. (2003). Role of environmental interventions in injury control and prevention. *Epidemiologic Reviews*, 25, 77-89.

Perrell, K.L., Nelson, A., Goldman, R.L., Luther, S.L., Prieto-Lewis, N., & Rubenstein, L.Z. (2001). Fall risk assessment measures: An analytic review. *Journal of Gerontology: Medical Sciences*, 56A(12), M761-M766.

Province, M.A., Hadley, E.C., Hornbrook, M.C., Lipsitz, L.A., Miller, J.P., Murlow, C.D., Ory, M.G., Sattin, R.W., Tinetti, M.E., & Wolf, S.L. (1995). The effects of exercise on falls in elderly patients: A preplanned meta-analysis of the FICSIT trials. Frailty and Injuries: Cooperative Studies of Intervention Techniques. *JAMA*, 273(17), 1341-1347.

Pynoos, J., Sabata, D., Abernethy, G.D., Alley, D., Nishita, C., & Overton, J. (2004). Prevention of falls at home: Best practices in home modification. In *Preventing falls in older Californians: State of art*. Archstone Foundation, Long Beach, CA, January 2003, revised October 2004.

Pynoos, J., Sabata, D., & Choi, I. (2004). The role of the environment in fall prevention at home and in the community. Prepared for the 2004 Falls Free: Promoting a National Falls Prevention Action Plan. Washington, DC.

RAND. (2003). *Fall prevention interventions in the Medicare population*. Prepared for U.S. Department of Health and Human Services. Centers for Medicare and Medicaid Services. Retrieved September 15, 2004, from http://www.cms.hhs.gov/healthyaging/fallspi.asp

Roberts, B.L. (2003). Falls: What a tangled web. *The Gerontologist*, 43(3), 598-601.

Rose, D.J. (2002). Promoting functional independence in older adults at risk for falls: The need for a multidimensional programming approach. *Journal of Aging and Physical Activity*, 10, 1-19.

Rose, D.J. (2002/2003). Results of intervention research: Implications for practice. *Generations*, 26(4), 60-65.

Rose, D.J. (2004). The role of exercise in reducing falls and fall-related injuries in older adults. Prepared for the 2004 Falls Free: Promoting a National Falls Prevention Action Plan. Washington, DC.

Rose, D.J., Abernethy, G.D., Castle, S.C., Horton, A., Missaelides, L.M., Nichols, J.F., & Vasquez, L. (2004). The California infrastructure and best practice models for fall prevention. In *Preventing falls in older Californians: State of art*. Archstone Foundation, Long Beach, CA, January 2003, revised October 2004.

Rubenstein, L.Z., Castle, S.C., Diener, D.D., Hooker, S.P., Jones, C.J., & Vasquez, L. (2004). Best practice interventions for fall prevention. In *Preventing falls in older Californians: State of art*. Archstone Foundation, Long Beach, CA, January 2003, revised October 2004.

Rubenstein, L.Z., & Josephson, K.R. (2002/2003). Risk factors for falls: A central role in prevention. *Generations*, 26(4), 15-21.

Rubenstein, L.Z., Kenny, R.A., Eccles, M., Martin, F., Tinetti, M.E., & AGS, BGS, AAOS Panel on Fall prevention. (2002/2003). Evidence-based guideline for fall prevention: Summary of the bi-national panel. *Generations*, 26(4), 38-41.

Salkeld, G., Cumming, R.G., O'Neil, E., Thomas, M., Szony, G., & Westbury, C. (2000). The cost effectiveness of a home hazard reduction program to reduce falls among older persons. *Australian and New Zealand Journal of Public Health*, 24(3), 265-271.

Shumway-Cook, A., Bruber, W., Baldwin, M., & Liao, O. (1997). The effect of multi-dimensional exercises on balance, mobility, and fall risk in community-dwelling older adults. *Physical Therapy*, 77(1), 46-57.

Steinberg, M., Cartwright, C., Peel, N., & Williams, G. (2000). A sustainable program to prevent falls and near falls in community dwelling older people: Results of a randomized trial. *Journal of Epidemiology and Community Health*, 54(3), 227-232.

Stevens, J.A. (2002/2003). Falls among older adults: Public health impact and prevention strategies. *Generations*, 26(4), 7-14.

Stevens, J.A. (2004). Falls among older adults–Risk factors and prevention strategies. Prepared for the 2004 Falls Free: Promoting a National Falls Prevention Action Plan. Washington, DC.

The National Council on the Aging. (2005). Falls free: Promoting a national falls prevention action plan: National action plan. Retrieved April 18, 2005 from [http://www.healthyagingprograms.org/resources/National%20Action%20Plan_Final.pdf]

Tideiksaar, R. (2001). Falls. In G.L. Maddox (Eds.), *The encyclopedia of aging* (3rd edition). (pp. 377-379). New York: Springer Publishing Company.

Tinetti, M.E. (2003). Preventing falls in elderly persons. *The New England Journal of Medicine*, 348(1), 42-49.

Tinetti, M.E., Baker, D.I., McAvay, G., Claus, E.B., Garrett, P., Gottschalk, M., Koch, M.L., Trainor, K., & Horwitz, R.I. (1994). A multifactorial intervention to reduce the risk of falling among elderly people living in the community. *The New England Journal of Medicine*, 331(13), 821-827.

Wolf, S.L., Barnhart, H.X., Kutner, N.G., McNeely, E., Coogler, C., & Xu, T. (1996). Reducing frailty and falls in older persons: An investigation of tai chi and computerized balance training. *Journal of the American Geriatrics Society*, 44(5), 489-497.

Wolf, S.L., Sattin, R.W., Kutner, M., O'Grady, M., Greenspan, A., & Gregor, R.J. (2003). Intense tai chi training and fall occurrences in older, transitionally frail adults: A randomized, controlled trial. *Journal of the American Geriatrics Society*, 51(12), 1693-1701.

Yates, S.M., & Dunnagan, T.A. (2001). Evaluating the effectiveness of a home-based fall risk reduction program for rural community-dwelling older adults. *The Journal of Gerontology: Medical Science*, 56A(4), M226-230.

Translating Evidence-Based Physical Activity Interventions for Frail Elders

Jennifer Wieckowski, MSG
June Simmons, LCSW

SUMMARY. The population shift to an older America has initiated a great deal of interest in the impact of evidence-based physical activity interventions on older adults. Physical activity for older adults has tremendous benefits and is recognized as one of the most powerful health interventions for improving seniors' ability to function and remain independent in the face of active health problems and yet the majority of all older adults remain largely sedentary. To date, few programs have been developed that apply these important research findings in physical activity to frail older adults living in the community. The purpose of this article is to review past and current trends addressing increasing physical activity in the frail elderly population at home. An exemplary model of integrating an evidence-based intervention into community-based care management programs is described. Barriers encountered when implementing evidence-based physical activity interventions with frail elderly at home and recommendations for future work in this area are discussed. *[Article copies available for a fee from The Haworth Document Delivery Service: 1-800-HAWORTH. E-mail address: <docdelivery@*

Jennifer Wieckowski and June Simmons are affiliated with the Partners in Care Foundation.

[Haworth co-indexing entry note]: "Translating Evidence-Based Physical Activity Interventions for Frail Elders." Wieckowski, Jennifer, and June Simmons. Co-published simultaneously in *Home Health Care Services Quarterly* (The Haworth Press, Inc.) Vol. 25, No. 1/2, 2006, pp. 75-94; and: *Evidence-Based Interventions for Community Dwelling Older Adults* (ed: Susan M. Enguídanos) The Haworth Press, Inc., 2006, pp. 75-94. Single or multiple copies of this article are available for a fee from The Haworth Document Delivery Service [1-800-HAWORTH, 9:00 a.m. - 5:00 p.m. (EST). E-mail address: docdelivery@haworth press.com].

KEYWORDS. Care management, frail older adults, physical activity, evidence-base, behavior change, brief negotiation, Stages of Change Model

INTRODUCTION

Current national initiatives are now shifting to a strong emphasis on the translation and adoption of evidence-based programs in the community. These types of programs are built on research findings that have been proven to work efficiently to improve the health and quality of life for individuals, groups, or communities. In today's competitive healthcare environment it is critical for providers to offer simple, cost-effective, and replicable programs that have been proven through credible research. Such programs should reliably generate positive results such as measurable improvement in health outcomes and increased client and provider satisfaction, thus resulting in higher quality services to the intended population. Integrating evidence-based programming into community-based health organizations must preserve the fundamental bridge of fidelity between the intervention researched and the new practice innovation, enabling providers to make more sophisticated decisions when planning, implementing and evaluating programs that have been established in tested models or interventions. Further information about the advantages of replicating evidence-based interventions can be found in the introduction article of this volume.

The population shift to an older America has initiated a great deal of interest in the impact of evidence-based physical activity interventions on older adults. Physical activity for older adults has tremendous benefits and is recognized as one of the most powerful health promotion interventions as well as improving seniors' ability to function and remain independent in the face of active health problems. The *Surgeon General's Report on Physical Activity and Health* (Center for Disease Control, 1996) concluded that Americans of all ages can substantially improve their health and quality of life by including moderate amounts of physical activity in their daily lives. To date, few if any programs have been developed and evaluated that apply these important research findings to in-home physical activity for older adults living in the community, especially very frail seniors. The work reported in this article targets a diverse, frail and low-income older population with an in-home evidence-based intervention to increase physical activity.

The purpose of this article, then, is to discuss strategies of bringing evidence-based research studies in physical activity into the care management practice setting, specifically in the community-based setting. First, it reviews the benefits of exercise that have been established in the research. Second, it provides a literature review of recent evidence-based exercise programs that have been shown to be effective for older adults. Third, it discusses an exemplary model of integrating an evidence-based physical activity intervention and behavior change counseling methods into the standard care plan of community based care management agencies serving the frailest older adult population living at home. This section discusses the barriers for translating evidence-based physical activity work into practice and discusses the early challenges, successes and lessons learned when modifying provider behavior to bring a tested vision into reality. Finally, this article provides recommendations for future work that needs to be done in this area.

BENEFITS OF EXERCISE

Interest in the benefits of physical activity has increased dramatically as a result of a wealth of recent studies that have documented that millions of Americans, especially older adults, suffer from chronic illnesses that may be prevented or better managed through participation in a structured physical activity program. A growing body of research overwhelmingly concludes that maintaining an active physical lifestyle in all adults, and including older adults, improves balance, prevents injurious falls, reduces symptoms of depression and pain, improves mental alertness and mood, reduces the risk of developing chronic diseases, moderates and promotes management of conditions such as high blood pressure, cholesterol, diabetes, and obesity, and improves the ability to function and stay independent in the face of chronic health problems such as lung disease or arthritis. The following section reports a summary of findings that demonstrate the benefits of exercise, thus establishing the urgency of developing methods for increased activity among the older adult population.

The role of physical activity contributing to psychological well-being in older adults has been explored in a number of studies in the past decade. These studies have found clear evidence that participation in a regular exercise program leads to improvement in mood, body image, cognitive functioning, well-being and self-esteem for older adults. It has been established that exercise promotes an antidepressant effect for depressed older adults, similar to psychological counseling or medication. Strawbridge, Deleger, Roberts, and Kaplan (2002) supported this argument with the finding that physical activity produces brain neurotransmitters which have a protective effect on depression. Babyak, Blumenthal, Herman, Khatri, Doraiswamy and Moore (2000) concluded that 16 weeks of exercise training is at least as effective as pharmacotherapy for depressive patients noting that systematic exercise also provided the patient with a sense of pride, personal mastery and positive self-regard. Many other studies support the conclusion that physical activity improves self-rated health, depression, morale, mental alertness and the psychological well-being of older adults (Ruuskanen & Ruoppila, 1995; Stathi, Fox & McKenna, 2002; Hill, Storandt & Malley, 1993).

Physical activity has also been identified in the literature as a strategy for increasing bone mass and bone mineral density and decelerating the development of osteoporosis and other chronic diseases in older adults. Results of a 1 year strength training program found that strength training had a positive effect on the risk factors for osteopenic fractures, including bone density, muscle mass, muscle strength, and balance (Nelson Fiatarone, Morganti, Trice, Greenberg, & Evans, 1994). Muscle strength, size and functional mobility can be re-built readily and with great benefit in the older frail population, even those in their nineties, through high resistance weight training exercises (Fiatarone, 1990). A 12 month randomized controlled trial found that exercise increased functional fitness, maintained bone mineral density, and improved spinal bone mass in osteopenic older adults (Bravo, Gauthier, Roy, Payette, Gaulin, Harvey et al., 1996). A positive effect was also found on psychological well-being, back pain intensity, and self-perceived health, suggesting how physical activity improves well-being and quality of life for older adults.

Physical activity also reduces the risk of debilitating hip fractures from injurious falls. Epidemiological studies suggest that active compared to sedentary older adults can minimize their risk of hip fracture through falls by improving muscle strength and balance. Even moderate levels of leisure activity, especially walking, have a protective effect against hip fractures in both older men and women (Kujala, Kaprio, Kannus, Sarna & Koskenvuo, 2000; Feskanich, Willett & Colditz, 2002). Physical activity may be a deterrent for falls and consequential fractures, although the type, frequency, intensity and duration of physical activity have not been established.

Perhaps even more persuasive are the results from a 12-year study involving 3,206 women and men over the age of 65 that show that even occasional physical activity extends the life expectancy among the elderly. Findings showed that those who were occasionally physically active had a 28 percent lower risk of all-cause mortality than those who were inactive. For those who were active once a week, the risk was over 40 percent lower for both men and women (Sundquist, Qvist, Sundquist & Johansson, 2004). These powerful results are indicative of the need for healthcare professionals and community-based organizations with ready access to frail elderly to encourage older adults to be more active, even occasionally.

Inactivity

Despite the scientific evidence that engaging in exercise has significant health benefits, the majority of all older adults remain largely sedentary. National data indicate only 31% of individuals aged 65-74 and only 23% of those 75 years and older engage in regular physical activity, defined as 20 minutes of moderate activity 3 or more days per week (AHRQ, 2003). This inactive lifestyle leads to loss of muscle and strength, which compromises balance and leads to falls, fractures, and other preventable complications. Inactivity is cited as one of the most disadvantageous factors contributing to impaired functioning and disability with age (King, Pruitt, Phillips, Oka, Rodenburg, & Haskell, 2000).

The underutilization of exercise among older adults is alarming, since this age group is the fastest growing population segment worldwide. It is estimated that by 2020 over 53.7 million older adults will be living in the United States, compared to 34.8 million in 2000 (U.S. Census Bureau, 2000). While many physiological changes are encountered in the body as people age, there is a growing body of evidence that weakened muscles, restricted movements, and stiff joints are not a normal part of aging for those who stay physically active. In response to a general national decline in activity levels Healthy People 2010 has established specific goals. One goal is to set physical activity goals for adults including both a decrease in the proportion of adults who engage in no leisure time physical activity and an increase in the proportion who engage regularly in moderate physical activity.

In efforts to improve the health of this at-risk population, the role of evidence-based physical activity interventions in slowing the progression of chronic diseases, maintaining independence, and improving the health status of older adults needs to become more of a national priority. Community-based organizations and their health care partners are potentially very effective vehicles for addressing the battle of inactivity among all ages, especially among the aging cohorts. In particular, care management programs have generally not addressed physical condition and physical activity as part of their formal assessment and care planning, largely as no clear and safe prescription for the frail was available. This article presents an early test of a solution to this challenge.

LITERATURE REVIEW

Physical activity has only recently been recognized in the research as an independent risk factor for all-cause mortality. Prior to 1980 it was uncommon for researchers to publish studies on exercise as a risk factor compared to other interventions such as smoking (Dunn & Blair, 2002). Since the 1990s the number of credible research studies that have been published concerning physical activity interventions has grown exponentially, creating an enormous body of evidence-based resources that could potentially be translated into practice. The research embraces a wide range of physical activity interventions that are appropriate for older adults of varying levels of fitness including strength, balance, flexibility and endurance exercises. There are many types of activities adults can take part in to improve their stamina, including walking, swimming, bicycling, stair climbing, dancing, weight training, and tai chi, to name a few.

While the most effective physical activity stimulus for gaining optimal health and functioning benefits in the older population living in the community has yet to be adequately defined or agreed upon via scientific consensus, most experts feels that a combination of endurance, strength and flexibility and balance activities are required (King, Rejeski & Buchner, 1998). Two major reviews in the literature of physical activity interventions describe the use of behavioral strategies aimed at promoting physical activity participation. One major review (King, Rejeski & Buchner, 1998) found 29 studies testing various physical activity interventions targeting older adults. Nearly half (45%) explicitly described specific behavioral, educational, social or cognitive strategies to elicit change. The most effective interventions included those that employed behavioral or cognitive-behavioral strategies as opposed to health education or instruction alone. Programs that used either a supervised home-based format or a combination of group- and home-based formats typically reported comparable or better physical activity adherence relative to programs that used a class or group format only. Ongoing telephone supervision was used in 7 studies and was shown to be an effective alternative to face-to-face on-site instruction, resulting in adherence rates over extended periods (up to 2 years) that were as good as or better than face-to-face instruction.

The benefits of a self-management program involving the client as the decision maker is also evident in the widely cited Arthritis Self-Management Program (Lorig, Mazonson & Holman, 1993). In this four year study arthritis patients attended a 6 session self-management class to set action plans and learn problem-solving skills to improve their self-efficacy and confidence to alter behaviors to reach a desired goal. Following the self-management course, the patients reported a mean reduction in pain symptoms of 20% whereas the comparison group did not demonstrate this improvement. The results of this study indicate that interventions involving the patient as the decision maker are more effective than traditional patient education approaches. This new behavior change paradigm involving a collaborative partnership between clinicians and clients may soon become a much more integral part of the healthcare system in supporting clients through the stages of change (Bodenheimer, Lorig, Holman & Grumbach, 2002).

Two well-designed studies focused on arthritis sufferers demonstrated that relevant intervention programs can be designed to promote long-term physical activity participation sufficient to reduce disability among this segment of the older adult population (King, Rejeski & Buchner, 1998). A study in 2001 assessed the effects of a multicomponent exercise program on basic daily functions and muscle strength in community-dwelling frail older adults. The intervention group demonstrated significant improvement in balance, muscle strength, walking function, and self-assessed functional ability compared to the control group (Worm, Vad, Puggaard, Stovring, Lauritsen, & Kragstrup, 2001).

Physical activity programs for older adults have been tested in many types of congregate settings, however, relatively few rigorous studies exist that focus specifically on in-home activities for frail, low-income community-dwelling older adults who account for the majority of multiple chronic conditions and disabilities. The in-home arena is an underdeveloped area in need of further research findings and sophisticated evaluation strategies. To date, in-home exercise interventions have been tried but it is rare to find evidence-based in-home work that has been evaluated sufficiently.

A well known research-based intervention with homebound seniors that can be integrated into the practice setting is The Well Elderly Study, the largest study ever conducted in the field of occupational therapy (Jackson, Carlson, Mandel, Zemke & Clark, 1998). This study demonstrated the benefits of preventive occupational therapy support for the elderly with the primary focus on "habit change." Study subjects were divided into three groups: one group received professionally-led occupational therapy, another group participated in social activities coordinated by non-professionals, and a third group had no programs at all. Findings showed that the participants in the occupational therapy group showed improvement in five of eight categories measured, while the control groups recorded declines across the board. The occupational therapists attempted to help participants better understand and appreciate the importance of meaningful activity in their lives, as well as teach them how to select and perform activities that would assist them in achieving a healthy and satisfying lifestyle.

A very significant study revealing the value of exercise for older adults was conducted by researchers Dr. Jessie Jones and Dr. Roberta Rikli (1999). This nationwide research project involving 7,183 older adults ages 60 to 94 in 21 different states examined the relationship between physical activity and functional mobility in later years and resulted in the Senior Fitness Test, the first standardized assessment tool which they developed for assessing the fitness levels of older adults. The study showed a markedly consistent pattern of decline in performance on the assessment parameters from age 60-94, revealing that in general there is an average decline in physical functioning of about 10% each decade between the ages of 60 and 90. This work serves as the foundation for the Healthy Moves for Aging Well intervention for homebound seniors enrolled in care management programs described in the next section. To date there needs to be pioneered evidence-based, safe, effective physical activity programs designed specifically for frail older adults in the home.

HEALTHY MOVES FOR AGING WELL–
AN EXEMPLARY MODEL

Many congregate community-based programs, although not always evidence-based, are currently available or being developed for well-elderly or elderly who are able to attend group activities either in senior centers or adult day health care centers. Few, if any, exercise programs have been developed that apply the important research findings in physical activity to frail, low-income and diverse elders for application in their homes. As a result, safety in the home for frail elders can be enhanced through evidence-based and function-linked movements that represent safe and appropriate "exercise" for this neglected, overlooked population. As society ages, it is essential to identify and disseminate simple, evidence-based physical activity programs targeted specifically for the frail older adult population in the home. This is a new emerging area of research that has been underdeveloped thus far.

An example of moving research findings into the community setting is the *Healthy Moves for Aging Well* physical activity program developed by Partners in Care Foundation in 2002 with guidance from a Los Angeles-based Regional Interdisciplinary Team of academic, clinical and community experts. This project was one of four model programs of the National Council on the Aging (NCOA) funded by the John A. Hartford Foundation. The *Healthy Moves* program, developed primarily for frail older adults receiving care management services, is an integrated model consisting of two evidence-based components described in detail below: a physical activity intervention modeled and adapted from the Senior Fitness Test work of Rikli and Jones (1999) and a lifestyle change counseling method called Brief Negotiation developed by behavior change experts Prochaska and DiClemente (1983). The integration of these two evidence-based models into community-based senior settings is an innovative partnership intended to increase the likelihood of older adults adopting a more active lifestyle.

Healthy Moves Physical Activity Component

The physical activity component of *Healthy Moves* is drawn from the evidence-based research-tested program the Senior Fitness Test, developed by Rikli and Jones (1999), which was previously described. This nationwide study tested the fitness levels of 7,183 older adults ages 60 to 94 using six exercise assessments linked to functional activities that are needed on a daily basis to live independently at home, including the chair stand, arm curl, two minute step-in-place, chair sit and reach, up and go, and scratch test. For the physical activity component of this evidence-based work, the developers of *Healthy Moves* collaborated with Rikli and Jones to select five seated and standing in-home exercises developed to improve the physical functioning of frail older adults with repetition. The seated exercises consist of arm curls, the seated step-in-place and the ankle point and flex. The standing exercises are for more advanced clients and include the chair stand and standing step-in-place. When appropriate, after mastery of the seated exercises, clinicians are trained to encourage their clients to graduate to the more advanced standing exercises that focus on balance, flexibility, endurance and stamina. Guidelines concerning the number of repetitions per movement are distributed to all participating clients and they are encouraged by their clinicians to do the movements three to five days per week.

The five *Healthy Moves* exercises were chosen and adapted from the Senior Fitness Test research by the experts because of their simplicity for the very frail population and their direct relationship to everyday movements and the specific muscles they target. For example, chair stands are important for getting out of a car and rising from a toilet or chair. By practicing exercises such as the seated or standing step-in-place and the ankle point and flex, clients ideally become more efficient with the exercises, build strength in the engaged muscles, increase flexibility, and even facilitate movements such as walking. The *Healthy Moves* are designed to help clients maximize their independence by giving them the strength to shop, hold grandchildren, get to the toilet, pour liquids to drink, and perhaps most importantly reduce the risk of falls (Table 1).

TABLE 1. How Do the Movements Apply to *My* Life?

Movements	Examples of Benefits	
Arm Curl	• Lifting/carrying laundry & groceries • Pouring a drink from a carton	• Upper body endurance & strength • Holding grandchildren
Ankle Point & Flex	• Increases ability to lift toes to avoid tripping on rugs, steps & curbs • Reduces fall risk	• Increases blood circulation to manage/prevent ankle swelling • Increases ankle flexibility
Seated Step-in-Place	• Getting to toilet • Walking in the home	• Shopping for groceries • Getting the mail
Standing Step-in-Place	• Getting to toilet • Walking outside to get ride	• Shopping for groceries • Getting the mail
Chair Stand	• Rising from a chair or toilet • Getting on & off public transportation	• Getting in & out of the car • Strengthen lower legs

HEALTHY MOVES INTEGRATED
BEHAVIOR CHANGE MODEL

The Brief Negotiation behavior change component of *Healthy Moves* is an evidence-based method that offers an innovative approach for clinicians to increase older adults' intrinsic motivation for making and sustaining changes in physical activity. The foundation of Brief Negotiation is modeled after the Stages of Change Model, also known as the Transtheoretical Model (Prochaska & DiClemente, 1983). The Stages of Change Model was established to recognize that people cycle through a series of stages as they strive to make and sustain successful lifestyle changes. The stages of change in relation to a physical activity program are precontemplation (client has no interest in starting to exercise), contemplation (client is thinking about starting but has made no plans), preparation (client is selecting to exercise), action (client starts exercising), and maintenance (client sustains new behavior) (Dunlap & Barry, 1999).

For the *Healthy Moves* program, the goal of the clinician is to assist the client's progress through the stages of change by using appropriate strategies that match the client's readiness to change. A simple method used in the *Healthy Moves* program for assessing a client's readiness to change involves a readiness ruler (Figure 1) scaled from 0 to 10 (higher numbers indicate greater readiness to change). The client is asked to select a number that best describes how ready s/he is to consider making a particular change. After understanding the client's current state of readiness, a variety of follow-up questions can be asked to help the client increase and strengthen intrinsic motivation (e.g., *What prompted you to pick a 4 and not a 1? What would it take for you to move from a 2 to a 5? How might your life be different if you begin exercising?*). This method, also known as "change talk," invites the client to make the arguments for change and ways of achieving it. This approach has been shown in the research literature to be related to whether a behavior change will actually occur (Bem, 1965; Amrhein et al., 2003).

The *Healthy Moves* Brief Negotiation training teaches clinicians that it is critical for them to understand and identify which stage their client is in before the physical activity intervention can be introduced and applied successfully. Traditional health care primarily focuses on imparting information–health professionals defining the problem, assessing client needs and prescribing supportive services. The reality is that receiving information and recommendations can assist clients to make more informed decisions, but they will not act on this information un-

FIGURE 1. How Ready Are You to Consider Increasing Your Physical Activity?

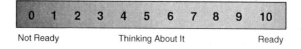

less they are motivated to do so. This finding has initiated a shift to a more collaborative partnership between the health professional and the client in which the client identifies the problem, sets goals and outlines an action plan to succeed. This approach teaches the client problem-solving skills and gives the client confidence and motivation to make decisions for a healthier lifestyle (Bodenheimer, Lorig, Holman, & Grumbach, 2002).

After it is clear that a client is motivated to make changes in activity levels, the clinician collaborates with the client to set goals and identify an achievable plan of action. Clinicians are trained to explore realistic goals with each client that can be accomplished through repetition and mastery of the *Healthy Moves* exercises (see Table 1). Goals frequently chosen by participating clients include walking in the home without falling, walking outside to get a ride, pouring a drink from a carton, rising from a toilet, and getting to the toilet on time.

The clinician also uses Brief Negotiation strategies to identify barriers for each client. Common barriers to adopting a physically active lifestyle among older adults include pain, poor health, educational level, weight, attitudinal barriers, fear of injury, social isolation, lack of time, information and motivation (Dunlap & Barry, 1999). An additional barrier for adherence to an exercise routine is knowledge of the importance of exercise. Physicians rarely impart advice about the value of exercise to their patients, thus undermining the importance of physical activity for older adults. A survey by the Centers for Disease Control and Prevention revealed that physicians inquired about diet and exercise less than one third of the time, a discouraging proportion given that physician advice is a powerful approach for initiating behavior change (MMWR & CDC, 1998).

Addressing these barriers and identifying specific personal goals that support changes have much more power to mobilize an individual to change behavior. When consistently incorporated into practice, Brief Negotiation strategies produce significant results for older adults: increased confidence in helping clients make and sustain changes in their lifestyles. In *Healthy Moves* this approach is incorporated to encourage increased physical activity levels, prevention of relapse into sedentary behavior, and subsequent improvements in patient satisfaction and health outcomes.

Integration of Healthy Moves into the Community

Integrating the physical activity work of Rikli and Jones with behavior change techniques enabled a model physical activity intervention adapted for frail seniors to be tested in community-based pilot sites in Los Angeles. The test sites were leading Medicaid Waiver care management sites in Los Angeles, known colloquially as the MSSP (Multipurpose Senior Services Program), including Huntington Hospital Senior Care Network, Jewish Family Service of Los Angeles, AltaMed Health Services Corporation and Partners in Care Foundation. These sites were chosen because geriatric care managers in these MSSP programs have ready access to frail elderly, trusting relationships and are already focused on maintaining their health status, delaying or preventing institutionalization, and improving linkages with medical and community resources. With no guidelines to suggest what to prescribe, physical activity has never been included in their standard care plans. Integration of a structured evidence-based physical activity program is compatible with the current goals and objectives of these programs.

A unique and favorable aspect of the *Healthy Moves* program is the involvement of motivational coaches who are recruited from the community to complement the role of the care managers in reinforcing behavior change. Dedicated, flexible and patient coaches with cultural and linguistic competency for the clients in the program are recruited and trained to call their assigned clients on a weekly basis to offer a form of social support, motivate the clients to adopt and maintain the recommended exercises, and to monitor each client's participation in the physical activity program. In some cases, the coaches actually visit the clients in the home and teach the *Healthy Moves* exercises.

In a three year pilot, care managers at the four select MSSP sites, with the assistance of trained community coaches, used Brief Negotiation strategies and motivational techniques to engage 49 clients in the *Healthy Moves* program. They assessed client functional ability using the Senior Fitness Test, taught a variety of safe and simple in-home exercises to improve strength and the overall health of the clients, and monitored client involvement in the program on a regular basis. The results of the *Healthy Moves* pilot incorporating these new tools were promising, with a high 76.2% client retention rate in the in-home exercise program after six months of participation. Improvements were seen in many of the clients, including a once-sedentary diabetic mono-lingual Lebanese client who lost 40 pounds, improved his blood-sugar levels, and became ineligible for the MSSP program because he became too healthy. Other clients also expressed enthusiasm for the program. A 71-year-old *Healthy Moves* participant suffering from congestive heart failure is now doing stretches, arm and leg lifts, and walking around her community pool. These favorable results of the pilot with four agencies clearly demonstrated the efficacy and value of the program for "able and willing" clients and have led to a broader application of this work.

The pilot demonstrated sufficient success with a small sample of 49 to lead to the current efforts to mainstream this innovation as a new practice standard in three California Medicaid Waiver care management settings, together serving up to 1,450 ethnically and linguistically diverse, low income and frail older adults on any given day. The test sites include Partners in Care Foundation MSSP South and two of the pilot sites, Jewish Family Service of Los Angeles and Huntington Hospital Senior Care Network. The work in this area is funded by the Archstone Foundation, The California Endowment and UniHealth Foundation and is recognized as one of the current United States Administration on Aging Evidence-based Prevention Programs for the Elderly.

The objective of the current project is to demonstrate the feasibility of changing care management practice to include behavior change strategies to improve levels of physical activity in frail elders. The success of *Healthy Moves* will be evaluated by pursuing the following three research questions: (1) Does the intervention change care manager behavior?; (2) Does the intervention change client behavior?; and (3) Does the intervention change the client's health outcomes? The targeted health outcomes include reduction of pain and depression, decrease in fear of falling and the number of injurious falls, and maintenance of or improvement in physical functioning. Finally, an overall goal of the program is to assure that the resulting physical activity program is cost effective, sustainable and replicable. The findings from this study will emphasize the importance of *Healthy Moves* for strengthening local, state and national care management programs with evidence-based approaches, increasing consumer choice through Brief Negotiation methods, and improving the quality of life of our most vulnerable seniors in America.

CHALLENGES, SUCCESSES AND LESSONS LEARNED

The pilot project of *Healthy Moves* facilitated the learning ground to discover and explore issues for supervisors, staff and clients in introducing an evidence-based physical activity program to culturally and linguistically diverse frail low income elderly. With great success as a pilot, multiple lessons have been learned. Principle among these was the recognition of how challenging it is to integrate change in any degree or form into existing community-based organizations, especially into care management programs requiring complex record-keeping with large client case loads.

In the pilot, the developers of *Healthy Moves* assumed that the primary challenge would be to motivate older adults to sustain participation in the exercise program. However, the pilot revealed that the majority of the clients actually had the interest and the time to devote to a simple exercise program, which is why the participation rate after six months of involvement was so high at 76.2%. The clients were pleased that the care managers and coaches believed they could increase their independence and quality of life by participation in an in-home exercise program. The extra attention and motivational support made the transition to an active lifestyle more appealing. In retrospect, the most challenging component of *Healthy Moves* was engaging the providers to adopt a new program into their established setting. While changing provider behavior is a difficult and complex task, there are solutions for achieving change in the practice setting despite the inherent barriers. The steps parallel the stages of individual behavior change.

One way to facilitate positive change in a setting is to assess the "readiness" of a practice setting to proceed with the implementation of an intervention, such as *Healthy Moves*. It is highly recommended that agencies utilize the Readiness Self-Assessment Tool, developed by a work group of the National Council on the Aging, when evaluating the readiness of a setting to introduce a new evidence-based intervention into practice (NCOA Center for Healthy Aging, 2004). This tool provides a framework for organizations and their partners to address key issues that indicate their potential for success with evidence-based programming. For example, before replicating the *Healthy Moves* program it is very important to develop strong relationships with supervisors and elicit buy-in from senior leadership and program administrators to ensure that the program receives programmatic and financial support and necessary time and attention by knowledgeable staff and agency leaders. Agency leaders need to evaluate the stability of their personnel and support staff before introducing a new standard of care into an agency which inherently disrupts the culture of an organization.

Following agreement from senior leadership and key partners to move forward with implementation, the next major barrier is attaining buy-in from the clinicians and providers who will be participating in the intervention. A key strategy for facilitating change is to involve the providers in the planning phase of the program. Joint planning with program staff, agency management and clinical staff helps identify valuable methods to modify the procedures for real world practice. Conducting focus groups with key players assists in identifying and developing methods that improve delivery of change counseling, exercise education, implementation, and maintenance within the care management model.

Another way to engage providers to participate in the *Healthy Moves* program is to design the intervention in a practical and feasible way to fit into their practice environment. The intervention, training time and procedural requirements must be simple and succinct. For example, in the pilot project the care managers attended extensive trainings to learn how to engage their clients in the *Healthy Moves* program. While the model was deemed effective and desirable by consumers and staff alike, some indicated it was too complex. The amount of training time for the pilot was valuable and valued, but would not be practical as a replicable model. The pilot revealed the need for judicious impact on care manager roles, time and workload. For future implementation, it was learned that the trainings must be streamlined to make adoption feasible for professionals and clients alike. A creative strategy invented by one care management setting was to build the *Healthy Moves* trainings into the regularly scheduled staff meetings to reduce additional time needed for trainings and to increase attendance at program meetings. Changing the practice standards, shifting staff responsibilities, and introducing a new standard of care almost always elicits a learning curve. However, reduced training has value for a more achievable level of change in the real world of care management with frail elders.

The intervention must also be designed to fit the practice environment of all involved parties. The intervention must be adaptable in order to make the program work. Flexibility and open-mindedness among care managers, supervisors, and staff are essential characteristics needed to facilitate change. Labor unions can also impact the change process. Staff members in community-based settings need training in validated and research-based physical activity approaches adapted for cultural differences, frailty, low income and in-home use. However, it is challenging to introduce a new practice standard into any agency. This is particularly true if the program faces other concurrent challenges such as shortages in staffing or a client-expansion phase in the program, complicating the clinical environment demands on staff. When integrating an intervention it must be noted that every agency is unique, therefore new innovations will be installed differently depending on staff personalities, site protocols and managerial expectations. Project staff and providers of care must recognize the benefits of gaining practice wisdom and insight when translating research findings into community-based settings. The intervention must be adaptable and designed conjointly among all involved parties.

Finally, marketing an intervention to clinicians in terms of value to their clients is a useful adoption strategy. Providers have a strong interest in improving the quality of life of their clients. For example, in the pilot the intervention was presented as a falls prevention strategy. A large majority of clients enrolled in Medicaid Waiver care management programs suffer from multiple injurious falls because of their frail condition and poor muscle strength in their lower extremities. As noted earlier in this article, a more active lifestyle may reduce the risk of falls and resulting injuries from a fall. Physical activity is also associated with reduced pain and depression and may increase the functional ability of older adults. Sharing client testimonials linked to these benefits in the form of videos, websites, newsletters, and presentations generates enthusiasm for adoption at the sites. The likelihood that a practice setting will adopt a new program into their standard of care weighs heavily on the way the program is marketed to the providers.

CONCLUSION

The importance of translating evidence-based research into community-based settings has been emphasized repeatedly as a current movement in health care. The *Healthy Moves* work is one of many exciting model programs that is modifying and adapting research findings, thus making it useful and practical for the practice setting. In fact, the *Healthy Moves* pilot was the first known attempt to bring evidence-based practice to the very frail and isolated homebound seniors enrolled in Medicaid-waiver care management programs in California.

As the *Healthy Moves* program is mainstreamed into select care management agencies it is expected that a great deal will be learned about the physical ability of Medicaid Waiver care management clients to engage in this program and the feasibility of mainstreaming this program into an entire agency while maintaining fidelity to the evidence-based model.

This approach is unique given that *Healthy Moves* utilizes existing staff and can be used during regularly scheduled visits with clients. Therefore the program holds tremendous promise of being cost-effective, culturally sensitive, and sustainable while improving the health of clients. The hope is that community based agencies can incorporate this model into care management programs without significant additional expense or time demands on staff. Demonstrating the pilot efforts to a full practice standard with a greater variety of clinicians and clients will be informative and enriching and will result in much greater depth in the training materials and supporting clinical tools for the second phase of the project as well as future replication.

Translating evidence-based work into the community setting and conducting a thorough and comprehensive evaluation of the impact of the program is a complex and challenging task. Interrupting the clinical culture with evidence-based innovations is a difficult process because change occurs at a gradual pace. However, testing and disseminating "best practices" and rising to the challenges and barriers that are presented is strategically important for strengthening the delivery of healthcare and social services in community-based settings. The work in this area is of much importance on a national level and the vision and diplomacy that has enabled community-settings to develop and test evidence-based disease prevention programs for older adults has only just begun.

REFERENCES

Agency for Healthcare Research and Quality. (2002). *Physical activity and older Americans: Benefits and strategies.* Agency for Healthcare Research and Quality and the Centers for Disease Control and Prevention. (Available online: *http://www.ahrq.gov/ppip/activity.htm*)

Amrhein, P., Miller, W., Yahne, C., Palmer, M., & Fulcher, L. (2003). Client commitment language during motivational interviewing predicts drug use outcomes. *Journal of Consulting and Clinical Psychology, 71*, 862-878.

Babyak, M., Blumenthal, J.A., Herman, S., Khatri, P., Doraiswamy, M., Moore, K. et al. (2000). Exercise treatment for major depression: Maintenance of therapeutic benefit at 10 months. *Psychosomatic Medicine, 62*, 633-638.

Bem, D. (1965). An experimental analysis of self-persuasion. *Journal of Experimental Social Psychology, 1*, 199-218.

Bodenheimer, T., Lorig, K., Holman, H., Grumbach, Kevin MD. (20 November 2002). Patient Self-management of Chronic Disease in Primary Care. *The Journal of the American Medical Association, 288*(19), 2469-2475.

Bravo, G., Gauthier, P., Roy, P., Payette, H., Gaulin, P., Harvey, M. et al. (1996). Impact of a 12-month exercise program on the physical and psychological health of osteopenic women. *Journal of the American Geriatrics Society, 44,* 756-762.

Centers for Disease Control and Prevention. (1996). *Physical activity and health: A report of the Surgeon General,* Atlanta, GA: C.D.C., 278.

Dunlap J., & Barry H. (1999). Overcoming exercise barriers in older adults. *The Physician and Sports Medicine, 27,* 69.

Dunn, A. & Blair, S. (2002). Translating evidence-based physical activity interventions into practice: The 2010 challenge. *American Journal of Preventive Medicine, 22,* 8-10.

Feskanich, D., Willett, W., & Colditz, G. (2002). Walking and leisure-time activity and risk of hip fracture in postmenopausal women. *Journal of the American Medical Association, 288,* 2300-2306.

Fiatarone, M., Assistant Professor at Harvard University, March 31, 1995. Active Living Institute Conference for Extended Vitality at Stanford University.

Graying of the US, 2000 (n.d.). *U.S. Census Bureau.* Retrieved June 1, 2005 from www.census.gov.

Hill, R.D., Storandt, M., & Malley, M. (1993). The impact of long-term exercise training on psychological function in older adults. *Journal of Gerontology, 48,* P12-P17.

Jackson, J., Carlson, M., Mandel, D., Zemke, R., & Clark, F. (1998) Occupation in lifestyle redesign: The well elderly study occupational therapy program. *American Journal of Occupational Therapy, 52,* 326-336.

King, A.C., Pruitt, L.A., Phillips, W., Oka, R., Rodenburg, A., & Haskell, W.L. (2000). Comparative Effects of Two Physical Activity Programs on Measured and Perceived Physical Functioning and Other Health-Related Quality of Life Outcomes in Older Adults. *Journal of Gerontology, 55A,* M74-M83.

King, A.C., Rejeski, W.J., & Buchner, D.M. (1998). Physical activity interventions targeting older adults: A critical review and recommendations. *American Journal of Preventive Medicine,* 15, 316-33.

Kujala, U.M., Kaprio, J., Kannus, P., Sarna, S., & Koskenvuo, M. (2000). Physical activity and osteoporotic hip fracture risk in men. *Archives of Internal Medicine, 160,* 705-708.

Lorig, K., Mazonson, P., & Holman, H. (1993). Evidence suggesting that health education for self-management in patients with chronic arthritis has sustained health benefits while reducing health care costs. *Arthritis Rheum, 36,* 439-446.

Missed opportunities in preventive counseling for cardiovascular disease: United States: 1995 (1998). *MMWR 47*(5), 91-95.

Nelson, M.E., Fiatarone, M.A., Morganti, C.M., Trice, I., Greenberg, R.A., & Evans, W.J. (1994). Effects of high-intensity strength training on multiple risk factors for osteoporotic fractures: A randomized controlled trial. *Journal of the American Medical Association, 272,* 1909-1914.

Prochaska, J.O., & DiClemente, C.C. (1983) Stages and Processes of Self-Change of Smoking: Toward an Integrative Model of Change. *Journal of Consulting and Clinical Psychology,* 51(3), 390-395.

Rikli, R. & Jones, J. (1999). Functional Fitness Normative Scores for Community-Re-siding Older Adults, Ages 60-94. *Journal of Aging and Physical Activity, 7,* 162-181.

Ruuskanen, J.M. & Ruoppila, I. (1995). Physical activity and psychological well-being among people aged 65 to 84 years. *Age and Ageing, 24,* 292-296.

Stathi, A., Fox, K., & McKenna, J. (2002). Physical activity and dimensions of subjective well-being in older adults. *Journal of Aging and Physical Activity, 10,* 76-92.

Strawbridge, W.J., Deleger, S., Roberts, R.E., & Kaplan, G.A. (2002). Physical activity reduces the risk of subsequent depression for older adults. *American Journal of Epidemiology, 156,* 328-334.

Sundquist, K., Qvist, J., Sundquist, J. & Johansson, S. (2004). Frequent and occasional physical activity in the elderly: A 12-year follow-up study of mortality. *American Journal of Preventive Medicine, 27,* 22-27.

U.S. Department of Health and Human Services. (November 2000). *Healthy People 2010: Understanding and improving health* (2nd ed.). Washington, DC: Government Printing Office.

Worm, C.H., Vad, E., Puggaard, L., Stovring, H., Lauritsen, J., & Kragstrup, J. (2001). Effects of a multicomponent exercise program on functional ability in community-dwelling, frail older adults. *Journal of Aging and Physical Activity, 9*(4), 414-424.

Moving Evidence-Based Interventions to Populations: A Case Study Using Social Workers in Primary Care

Scott Miyake Geron, PhD
Bronwyn Keefe, MSW, MPH

SUMMARY. This article describes a study to expand a proven evidence-based practice for depression to a population-based intervention for frail older adults. Problem-Solving Therapy (PST) has been proven effective in reducing depression and other mental health conditions in cognitively intact adults in many studies. The current study employs a randomized controlled trial to test the effectiveness of a social work intervention for frail older adults that uses PST to address depression and other psychosocial issues. The intervention employs Master's trained social workers integrated into a large primary care practice. The study population is comprised of home-dwelling older adults with multiple chronic conditions, a recent history of unnecessary hospitalizations, and no more than mild cognitive impairment. *[Article copies available for a fee from The Haworth Document Delivery Service: 1-800-HAWORTH. E-mail*

Scott Miyake Geron is Director and Principal Investigator and Associate Professor of Social Welfare Policy and Research, and Bronwyn Keefe is Assistant Director and Co-Principal Investigator, both at the Institute for Geriatric Social Work, Boston University School of Social Work, 232 Bay State Road, Boston, MA 02215.

[Haworth co-indexing entry note]: "Moving Evidence-Based Interventions to Populations: A Case Study Using Social Workers in Primary Care." Geron, Scott Miyake, and Bronwyn Keefe. Co-published simultaneously in *Home Health Care Services Quarterly* (The Haworth Press, Inc.) Vol. 25, No. 1/2, 2006, pp. 95-113; and: *Evidence-Based Interventions for Community Dwelling Older Adults* (ed: Susan M. Enguídanos) The Haworth Press, Inc., 2006, pp. 95-113. Single or multiple copies of this article are available for a fee from The Haworth Document Delivery Service [1-800-HAWORTH, 9:00 a.m. - 5:00 p.m. (EST). E-mail address: docdelivery@haworthpress.com].

Available online at http://www.haworthpress.com/web/HHC

doi:10.1300/J027v25n01_06

KEYWORDS. Evidence-based practice, Problem-Solving Therapy (PST), social work, primary care, depression, psychosocial issues, and older adults

Evidence-based practice has been defined as the "conscientious, explicit and judicious use of current best evidence" (Kerridge, Lowe, & Henry, 1998) and is quickly emerging as one of the most important movements to improve the efficiency and effectiveness of clinical care. Initially applied to medicine (Cochrane, 1972; Sackett, Rosenberg, Muir Gray, Haynes, & Richardson, 1996; West, 2000), evidence-based practice is now influencing fields as diverse as nursing (Sackett et al., 1996), psychiatry (Drake et al., 2001), and social work (Gambrill, 2001). Evidence-based practice informs clinical efforts through a number of research approaches (Sackett et al., 1996; Rychetnik, Hawe, Waters, Barratt, & Frommer, 2004), such as evidence-based reviews, meta-analyses, expert opinion, and randomized controlled trials (Bartels et al., 2002). Proponents in medicine have claimed that by incorporating the best evaluated methods of health care, evidence-based practice leads to improvements in clinicians' knowledge, teaching methods, communication with patients, and, most important, patient outcomes (Kerridge et al., 1998).

One of the challenges in evidence-based practice is to generalize the results of the clinical intervention to populations or conditions different from those originally targeted (Flaherty, Morley, Murphy, & Wasserman, 2002). Typically, in medical practice, where much of the work so far has been done, research on evidence-based clinical practice focuses on specific patient conditions or illnesses like COPD, or congestive heart failure, using defined protocols and trained health professionals, typically nurses or physicians (Lisansky & Clough, 1996; Kunik et al., 2001). The narrow focus of the protocols on specific patient diseases or conditions allows for more precise testing (in general, the more limited, focused, and standardized the intervention, the easier it is to control in a statistical sense, and the easier it is to evaluate). From a research point of view, this type of specification makes sense, as it eliminates many confounding factors. The gradual build-up of evidence in support of a particular clinical practice occurs when the same procedure is used to address the same problem or condition in a related, but different patient or client population (e.g., a different age group), while still following the precise protocols originally found to be effective. One factor limiting the testing of evidence-based clinical practice is the common reluctance of the originators of the protocol to change the parameters considered essential to the integrity or success of the original intervention.

From a policy point of view, this process of developing evidence in support of a clinical intervention is problematic for two reasons. First, the narrow focus of most clinical studies, while desirable from a research point of view, may work against the interests of policy change, since policy makers are more likely to support general programs that address multiple patient conditions or illnesses (e.g., Medicaid waiver programs and Medicare Home Health Programs), rather than clinical interventions that are specific to a particular disease or condition (Kane, Kane, & Ladd, 1998). This is especially true if the desired aim is to expand reimbursement options to support the clinical intervention. Second, the strict adherence to original protocols tested in clinical studies often makes it hard to expand the focus of these interventions to populations or conditions that would make the interventions attractive to policy makers. The paradox is that the needs of research for specificity, control, and interventions focused on particular patient diseases or conditions are at cross purposes with the needs of policy for research findings that show clinical interventions that are population-based, generalizable across different patient groups and multiple conditions, and amenable to administration by different professionals.

This paper presents an example of a study that attempts to address the needs of both research and policy in the evaluation of an evidence-based practice. This study builds upon an evidence-based model of care with the goal of expanding this model to a broader population base. At the core of this research intervention is the use of Problem-Solving Therapy (PST). In a review of evidence-based practices in geriatric mental health, PST was identified as an effective treatment for geriatric depression (Bartels, Haley, & Dums, 2002). Williams et al. (2000) conducted a large clinical trial comparing the effects of paroxetine hydrochloride, PST, or placebo with adults over 60 who had minor depression or dysthymia. The authors found that both paroxetine and PST improved mental health functioning when compared to placebo. The effectiveness of PST has been evaluated in multiple randomized controlled trials in community settings and the most salient findings from these studies is that, in addition to depression, PST is an effective treatment for many other mental health conditions (Hegel & Arean, 2003; Catalan et al., 1991; Mynors-Wallis et al., 2000; Dowrick et al., 2000). Problem-solving therapy has also been successfully used in interventions with caregivers of medically and cognitively impaired elders (Teri, Logsdon, Uomoto, McCurry, 1997; Grant, Elliott, Giger Newman, Bartolucci, 2001). PST has been found to be effective in treating major depression in younger adults, older adults, medical patients, and mildly retarded adults (Alexopoulos & Chester, 2003). A recent study conducted by Alexopoulos, Raue, & Arean (2003) found PST to be more effective than supportive therapy in reducing depressive symptoms and disability in elderly patients with executive dysfunction. Furthermore, PST has been found to be an effective treatment for a variety of behavioral disorders, including schizophrenia (Liberman, Eckman, & Marder, 2001; Medalia, Revheim, & Casey, 2001), childhood autism (Bernard-Opitz, Sriram, & Nakhoda-Sapuan, 2001), attention deficit disorder (Barkley, Edwards, Laneri, Fletcher, & Metevia, 2001), and substance abuse (Zanis, Coviello, Alterman, & Appling, 2001). PST has also been found to be effective in the self-management of medical conditions, such as diabetes (Cook, Herold, Edidin, & Briars, 2002), cancer (Schwartz et al., 1998; Allen, Shah, Nezu, Nezu, Ciambrone, & Hogan, 2002; Sahler et al., 2002), and chronic pain (Ahles, Seville, Wasson, Johnson, Callahan, & Stukel, 2001). PST has served as a primary component for multifaceted interventions aimed at reducing depression among older adults. The Hartford Foundation funded IMPACT study was a national multi-site study that examined the effects of a multifaceted, stepped care intervention on older adults with major depression and dysthymia. About 1,800 primary care patients were randomized to usual care or to the IMPACT intervention that provided education, care management, and antidepressant medication or PST (Unutzer, 2002). This multifaceted model of care was effective in reducing depression among older adults (Unutzer, 2002). Enguidanos, Davis, and Katz (2003) conducted a clinical trial with depressed older adults in a geriatric care management program using a stepped care treatment program that included PST and/or antidepressant medication, and found that the symptoms of depression lessened in older adults who received the integrated treatment. In conclusion, PST has been shown to be an effective evidence-based treatment for depression and other mental health disorders in older adults.

This study employs a randomized controlled trial (RCT) to test a social work intervention with frail older adults in primary care. The intervention is designed to reduce unnecessary hospitalization and improve patient outcomes. The study population is a group of home-dwelling older adults with multiple chronic conditions, a recent history of unnecessary hospitalizations, and no more than mild cognitive impairment. A master's-level social worker located in a primary care office is conducting the intervention. The main goal of the study is to test the effectiveness of a social work intervention in a primary care setting. Another goal of the study is to expand the evidence-based practice model in four respects in order to meet broader policy objectives of the study: (1) expand the target population to include a frail older population with multiple chronic illnesses, a group of interest to policy makers because of its high medical-utilization costs; (2) expand targeted outcomes to include psychosocial issues in addition to depression; (3) alter the intervention team to include master's-level social workers rather than nurses; and (4) expand the intervention protocol to include care management, a potentially reimbursable component in the new Medicare legislation.

IMPORTANCE OF INTEGRATING SOCIAL WORKERS INTO A PRIMARY CARE SETTING

The vast majority of older people who receive health care obtain it in the context of a visit to their primary care provider. The rising costs of inpatient care and incentives within the Medicare prospective payment system combine to motivate health care providers to find outpatient alternatives to inpatient treatment (Bodenheimer, Wagner, & Grumbach, 2002). Advances in technology and a new generation of pharmacological advances also allow outpatient treatment of more illnesses (physical and psychological) that formerly could only be treated in the hospital, and the primary care practice often is that outpatient setting.

The primacy of primary care as a location of health care for frail older adults makes it an ideal setting in which to identify and treat mental health and psychosocial problems among this population. Declines in mental health funding, and the proven reluctance of elders, relative to younger adults, to seek specialty mental health services (Unutzer, 2002) are additional factors that suggest primary care as an appropriate setting for addressing mental health and psychosocial issues. Moreover, the link between mental health and physical health are now well established. Untreated mental illness has been associated with increased health care costs, increased use of primary care visits and consultations, and longer hospital stays, even after adjusting for pre-existing medical comorbidities (Unutzer, 1999). Recent studies have shown significant improvements in related care and patient outcomes for older adults when depression treatments are integrated into a primary care practice (Oxman & Dietrich, 2002).

OVERVIEW OF THE INTERVENTION

At the core of the study's social work intervention is the use of intensive Problem-Solving Therapy (PST), as noted, a validated behavioral change approach shown to be effective in treating depression. Similar to other behavioral change methods (Lorig & Laurin, 1985; Lorig, 1993; Wagner, Austin, & Von Korff, 1996), PST teaches patients to address current life difficulties by reducing large problems to smaller sections and identifying specific steps toward positive change (D'Zurilla & Nezu, 1987). Theoretically, PST incorporates key elements of social cognitive theory (Bandura, 1986; Bandura, 1997) but also has roots in empowerment models of practice (Anderson, Funnell, Butler, Arnold, Fitzgerald, & Feste, 1995), motivational interviewing (Botelho & Skinner, 1995; Miller, 1996; Schilling, El-Bassel, Finch, Roman, & Hanson, 2002), behavioral change theory (Wagner, Austin, & Von Korff, 1996; Wagner, Austin, Davis, Hindmarsh, Schaefer, & Bonomi, 2001), and social work problem-solving methods (Perlman, 1957). Particularly salient is Bandura's concept of self-efficacy, which refers to the individual's belief that he or she can actually perform an action or behave in a certain way. This belief is strongly related to the successful outcome of the individual's action.

Primary care practices are well positioned to improve the health outcomes of their frail elderly patients by providing physical and mental health care in a community setting as part of their regular regimen. Frail elders with chronic illness are frequent patients at primary care physician offices, often with a range of psychosocial and physical problems, from social isolation to minor depression to dementia. And, while recent studies have shown significant improvements in related care and patient outcomes for older adults when depression treatments are integrated into a primary care practice (Oxman & Dietrich, 2002), these busy medical offices do not generally have the capacity to provide such treatment or to coordinate care or link patients to other services that may enhance their independent living and improve health outcomes. Integrating a social work intervention that includes PST and care management into primary care settings is one way to address fragmentation among service delivery systems. For a number of reasons, then, an evidence-based intervention addressing depression and other psychosocial issues is sorely needed.

A brief, protocolized care management intervention is being provided to patients in the intervention group who decline to participate in PST. In line with the process of PST, the social worker will assist the patient in generating a problem list, and will then help the patient select a problem and identify the necessary steps to resolve the problem. The social worker will encourage the patient to identify possible solutions and will assist in providing solutions when needed. Unlike PST, these sessions will involve direct assistance from the social worker and will address problems defined by the physician, the patient, or the social worker. Patients may choose to enroll in PST at any point during the case management sessions, but a limit of eight visits with the patient (for care management or PST or both) will be provided.

If an emergent issue is identified at the onset of the case or at any time during the intervention, the social worker will stop the PST and provide immediate assistance in addressing that issue before resuming the intervention steps. Emergent issues are defined as any situation where the patient is at risk for imminent harm, self-inflicted or from others. In these cases, and contrary to the PST intervention, the social worker may work with the patient's family or caregiver independent of the patient to provide limited assistance to address the emergent issues. This assistance could include providing referrals or providing help in locating resources.

Participants randomly assigned to the intervention group will be offered up to eight PST sessions with the social worker, with each session averaging about 45 minutes. At session four, the social worker will determine if the patient meets discharge criteria, which is defined as the successful resolution of two problems during PST sessions plus independent application and resolution of at least two problems outside of the sessions. If patients do not meet discharge criteria, up to four additional PST sessions are provided. PST sessions are conducted either in the primary care office or at the patient's home (if the patient is unable to get to the office), with follow-up sessions typically completed by telephone. Patients are strongly encouraged to come to the primary care clinic for social work services when possible. Some patients experience mobility and transportation problems requiring the social worker to make home visits to conduct the intervention.

DESIGN OF THE STUDY

This study is designed as a randomized controlled trial. Eligible respondents are randomly assigned to either the social work intervention group or the control group (who receive usual care). Data for the clinical trial is being gathered through in-person interviews (by phone or face-to-face) with experimental and control group subjects.

The key components of the intervention are the following:

- Place a master's-level social worker in a large primary care office.
- Build a patient-centered, collaborative, interdisciplinary primary-care team by placing the social worker at the office, and involving the person in the care of patients with physicians, nurses, and other health care professionals.
- Train master's-level social workers to use PST and care management to address depression and other psychosocial issues.
- Identify a diverse cohort of frail, older patients experiencing difficulties in managing their multiple chronic conditions (as evidenced by unscheduled hospital admissions or emergency room visits) and assess the impact of PST and care management on the patients' functioning, depression, and other health outcomes as well as service utilization and cost.
- Conduct a randomized controlled trial to test the social work intervention with a sample of frail older adults with multiple chronic conditions.
- Collect data from patients in the study in control and treatment groups at the first encounter, at four months, and at 12 months, and perform statistical analysis comparing treatment subjects to controls.

Research Site. This intervention is being conducted in a primary care clinic of a managed care organization in a large metropolitan area. The medical office has approximately 16 primary care physicians who serve an average of 30,000 patients, approximately 15 percent, or 4,500, of whom are 65 or older. The medical office offers family medicine, gynecology, internal medicine, laboratory, mammography, member health education, pediatrics, and a pharmacy.

Subjects. An estimated 524 subjects will be enrolled in the study over a two-year period. Subjects will reflect the overall enrollment of the managed care organization's members: approximately 40 percent of the members are Latino, 13 percent Asian, 32 percent white, and 14 percent African American, and many of the senior members have income levels below the poverty line.

Subjects must meet the following criteria to be eligible to participate in the study:

- Current patients at the medical office
- 65 years of age or older
- Diagnosed as having two or more chronic medical conditions

- Documented as having at least one emergency room visit or unscheduled hospital admission in the past 6 months
- Cognitively intact (as measured by a score of 7 or less on the Short Portable Mental Status Questionnaire)

The primary target population for this intervention is patients who have a history of high health care utilization. The rationale for choosing this group is to target those patients who are incurring the highest costs for utilization in order to see the greatest change. The rationale for requiring at least one visit to the emergency room or hospital in the past 6 months is to capture a frail population who are demonstrating difficulty in managing their condition. Finally, patients must be cognitively intact in order to participate in PST because the intervention is based on cognitive behavioral theory, which is inappropriate for patients with severe cognitive impairment.

This study is using master's-level social workers to provide PST and care coordination instead of nurses or depression clinical specialists, who have been used in the past (Saur et al., 2002; Oishi et al., 2003) for a number of reasons. First, recent reviews suggest that social workers possess specialized training in providing psychosocial assessment, care management, and information and referral services, all of which are critical components of the proposed intervention. Also, a growing number of empirical studies are using social workers to test psychosocial and care management interventions in the context of primary care because recent randomized clinical trials employing social workers to provide such interventions have found social workers to be effective in reducing the following: (1) emergency visits (Rosen, Proctor, & Staudt, 1999; Claiborne & Vandenburgh, 2002); (2) length of hospital stay (Williams, Williams, Zimmer, Hall, & Podgorski, 1987; Nikolaus, Specht-Leible, Bach, Oster, & Shlierf, 1999; Claiborne & Vandenburgh, 2002); (3) hospital admissions (Rubin, 1992; Rosen, 1999); (4) overall costs per patient (Williams et al., 1987; Nikolaus et al., 1999; Rosen, 1999); and (5) nursing home placement (Williams et al., 1987; Nikolaus et al., 1999). A number of RCTs have also noted increases in self-reported indicators of quality of life among elder patients receiving social work interventions (Morrow-Howell, Proctor, & Dore, 1998; Burns, Nichols, Martindale-Adams, & Graney, 2000; Rizzo & Rowe, 2003).

The integration of the social worker into the primary care practice is an important part of the study. The medical office has provided office space for the social worker to meet privately with the patient. Meeting with the patient within the primary care setting will do the following:

(1) increase exposure of the clinical care team to the social worker; (2) provide increased opportunities for the social worker to interact with the primary care team; and (3) allow the patient to interact with the social worker within a familiar environment. The social worker's involvement in the primary care office is being documented through daily activity logs of encounters with primary care physicians, including number of interactions with patients and staff, and course of action.

CONCEPTUAL MODEL, STUDY HYPOTHESES, AND VARIABLES OF INTEREST

The relationship among the variables of interest is depicted in Figure 1 relating to the hypothesized effects of the PST and care management intervention. Three sets of outcomes are hypothesized: (a) Patient; (b) Patterns of Care; and (c) Provider Behavior.

The following hypotheses are being tested by the intervention (shown in circles in Figure 1):

1. Frail older adults with multiple chronic conditions receiving the Social Work in Primary Care intervention will demonstrate improved self-efficacy to perform specific targeted self-management actions as compared to those receiving usual care.
2. Depressed, frail older adults with multiple chronic conditions receiving the Social Work in Primary Care intervention will have lower rates of depression as compared to those receiving usual care.
3. Frail older adults with multiple chronic conditions receiving the Social Work in Primary Care intervention will experience fewer declines in physical functioning as compared to those receiving usual care.
4. Frail older primary care practice patients receiving the Social Work in Primary Care intervention will report increased satisfaction with the services they receive as compared to those receiving usual care.
5. Frail older adults with multiple chronic conditions receiving the Social Work in Primary Care intervention will be less likely to use acute care services as compared to those receiving usual care, as demonstrated by fewer emergency room visits and hospital admissions.

6. The cost-utility ratio (CUR) for the Social Work in Primary Care Intervention is expected to be less than $50,000/quality adjusted life years (QALY).
7. Frail older adults with multiple chronic conditions receiving the Social Work in Primary Care intervention will be less likely to be admitted to a nursing facility in the 12 months following study enrollment as compared to those receiving usual care.

As shown in Figure 1, patient characteristics are independent variables that will be examined for their influence on the intervention. These characteristics include the participant's age, gender, marital status, ethnicity, education level, income level, diagnoses, living arrangement, social support, and cognitive status. Living situation will capture both types of housing and household composition. Social support will be assessed by asking for the patient's primary caregiver. Ethnicity refers to African American, Latino, Asian-Pacific Islander, Caucasian, Native American, other, or unknown.

As noted, cognitive status is important because PST has been proven to be most effective with cognitively intact clients, and, in this study, patients with moderate or severe cognitive impairment will be excluded from participation. Cognitive status is being assessed with the Short Portable Mental Status Questionnaire (Pfeiffer, 1975). The aim of PST and other behavior change strategies is to increase the participant's self-efficacy to manage his/her chronic illnesses. Thus, the intervention is expected to have a direct effect on self-efficacy and problem-solving skills, which, when generalized by the patient to other health and social problems, will lead to the principal outcomes in the study.

Patient outcomes are being measured using the Physical Functioning Domain from the SF-36 (Ware & Sherbourne, 1992; Ware, Kosinski, & Keller, 1996; Katz, Larson, Phillips, Fossel, & Liang, 1992), the Geriatric Depression Scale Short Form (Sheikh & Yesavage, 1985), a Patient Satisfaction Measure developed by the study's principal investigator, and the European Quality of Life Scale (Anonymous, 1990). The instruments have been pre-tested by research assistants to ensure face validity and comprehension. The research assistants conducted test interviews among geriatric care managers in the medical office, professionals who are experts on the target population and in the bio-psychosocial issues experienced by this population. The instrument was then pre-tested with members of the target population to further assess appropriateness and clarity of the instrument.

The Social Work in Primary Care intervention is expected to have an indirect effect on patterns of health care utilization, as a result of im-

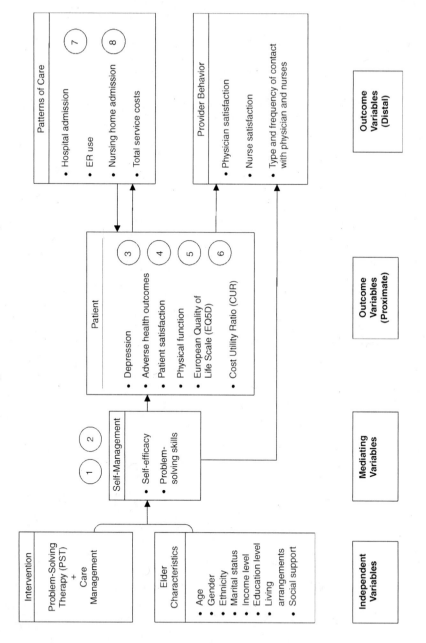

FIGURE 1. Causal Model of Social Work in Primary Care Intervention

proved self-efficacy and problem-solving skills among patients, and subsequent improvements in patient outcomes. It is also anticipated that reductions in unnecessary health care utilization may have a reciprocal beneficial effect on patient outcomes.

The medical office maintains accurate and extensive clinical records for all members, and these records will be used to obtain utilization variables of interest in this study for both treatment and control patients. The key utilization variables that will be analyzed are emergency room visits, inpatient hospital days, skilled nursing facility days, physician visits, and home health visits. To assess cost-effectiveness of the intervention, cost-utility ratios (CURs), a form of cost-effectiveness, will be assessed. CURs are based on the QALY utility scale (0 = death, 1 = optimal health) as measured by the EuroQol (Coons, Rao, Keininger, & Hays, 2000; Lawrence & Fleishman, 2004; Sapin, Fantino, Nowicki, & Kind, 2004). One major advantage of CURs is that they provide an unofficial standard for "worthwhile" interventions–$50,000 per QALY. Ratios below that level are considered to be cost-effective and are likely to be funded by policy makers.

The Social Work in Primary Care intervention is expected to have a direct effect on provider behavior, as seen in improved satisfaction of the PCP and other key staff (see Figure 1). This effect will be measured in the following ways: (1) focus groups; (2) physician and nurse contact log; (3) social work logs; and (4) physician and nurse satisfaction questionnaires.

DATA COLLECTION

Data is being collected from patients in the control and treatment groups at the first encounter, at four months, and at 12 months. Trained master's-level research assistants are conducting the screening telephone interview, the baseline assessment, and all follow up assessments. This information is being collected via participant self-reports. Diagnoses are verified through the medical office's electronic patient records. The screening interview takes approximately 5-10 minutes, while the baseline and follow-up interviews will last approximately 20-30 minutes. Baseline measures are conducted via telephone within 48 hours of receipt of signed informed consent. Follow-up measures also being collected via telephone surveys at four and 12 months. In addition, medical service use data will be collected from the medical office databases described above.

This study has received IRB approval from all participating institutions. Patients identified as eligible via telephone screening will receive an in-depth explanation of the study by the research assistant. Upon arrival at the clinic for their usually scheduled appointment, the eligible patients are given an informed consent sheet describing study participation. The patients are asked to review the consent form before their physician arrives in the office. Patients interested in participating in the study are asked to sign an informed consent form that will have been carefully reviewed with them by the research assistant, with any questions answered by their physician.

CONCLUSION

With a future of increasing public costs for health care, fragmentation in the system of care, and pressures on health care providers to treat patients on an outpatient basis and in ambulatory settings, the development of cost-effective interventions to address multiple chronic illnesses and psychosocial needs of frail older adults in primary care is urgently needed. One promising approach is the integration of evidence-based interventions addressing psychosocial issues in primary care and the use of ancillary services such as care coordination and care management.

Evidence-based medicine is defined as "the integration of best research evidence with clinical expertise and patient values" (Tickle-Degnen & Bedell, 2003). For depression, a growing body of research on effective psychosocial treatments is available, yet few older adults receive evidence-based treatments for depression in primary care (Unutzer, 2002), and little is known about the effectiveness of expanding these evidence-based models to address issues other than depression among older adults. Guidelines for treating mental health issues have been written and provided to primary care practices, and yet many of these illnesses are still untreated. In addition, current primary care providers lack the time and training to address depression and other psychosocial issues. Critics of evidence-based medicine believe that its practice may require time and resources not available to busy clinicians (Straus & McAlister, 2000). The different priorities and capacities of primary care providers, on the one hand, and mental health providers, on the other, in serving the aging population can further complicate the implementation of evidence-based treatments (Bartels et al., 2002). For this reason, it makes sense to have an interdisciplinary team working together to apply evidence-based practice, within the specific disciplines of each team member.

This article summarizes a research study that has integrated a social worker within the primary care setting in order to expand upon a tested evidence-based practice for depression to a population-based social work intervention, which also includes care management. The aims of the study are to maintain fidelity with the original core components of the intervention, but to expand its scope to increase the chances of making an impact on public policy. Some of the challenges faced in translating this evidence-based model for a broader population include: (1) fine-tuning the eligibility criteria to target a large group of cognitively intact frail elders who can benefit from PST; (2) modifying the discharge criteria to accurately document the successful completion of PST; and (3) identifying the criteria for successful adaptation by practicing social workers for an intervention employed generally by nurse practitioners or mental health specialists. These challenges illustrate the obstacles that are necessary to overcome when expanding evidence-based practices to different populations and settings. Furthermore, it shows that it is necessary to be flexible when embarking on new trials that are aiming to expand the scope of proven evidence-based practices, and demonstrates the potential difficulties in attempting to exactly replicate the procedures and/or findings of previous studies to these different populations. It is important to address these challenges and move towards the ultimate goal of impacting policy. Finally, through wider application of evidence-based practices among older adults, this study aims to impact policy by (1) demonstrating that interventions using geriatric social workers are as effective as or more effective than other interventions using more expensive workers (such as nurses or physicians); and (2) documenting that integrating social workers in primary care leads to improved patient outcomes, increased provider satisfaction, and cost-effective care.

REFERENCES

Ahles, T., Seville, J., Wasson, J. H., Johnson, D., Callahan, E., & Stukel, T. (2001). Panel-based pain management in primary care: A pilot study. *Journal of Pain Symptom Management, 22*(1), 584-590.

Alexopoulos, G. S., & Chester, J. G. (1992). Outcomes of geriatric depression. *Clinics in Geriatric Medicine, 8*(2), 363-376.

Alexopoulos, G. S., Raue, P., & Arean, P. (2003). "Problem-solving therapy versus supportive therapy in geriatric major depression with executive dysfunction." *Am. J Geriatric Psychiatry* 11(January-February, 2003): 46-52.

Allen, S., Shah, A., Nezu, A., Nezu, C., Ciambrone, D., & Hogan, J. (2002). A problem-solving approach to stress reduction among younger women with breast carcinoma: A randomized controlled trial. *Cancer, 94*(12), 3089-3100.

Anderson, R. M., Funnell, M. M., Butler, P. M., Arnold, M. S., Fitzgerald, J. T., & Feste, C. C. (1995). Patient Empowerment: Results of a randomized controlled trial. *Diabetes Care, 18*(7), 943-949.

Anonymous. (1990). EuroQoL–a new facility for the measurement of health-related quality of life. The EuroQol Group. *Health Policy, 16*(3), 199-208.

Bandura, A. (1986). *Social foundations of thought and action: A social cognitive theory.* Englewood Cliffs, New Jersey: Prentice-Hall.

Bandura, A. (1997). *Self-Efficacy: The exercise of control.* New York: W.H. Freeman & Co.

Barkley, R. A., Edwards, G., Laneri, M., Fletcher, K., & Metevia, L. (2001). The efficacy of problem-solving communication training alone, behavior management training alone, and their combination for parent-adolescent conflict in teenagers with ADHD and ODD. *Journal of Consulting & Clinical Psychology, 69*(6), 926-941.

Bartels, S. J., Dums, A. R., Oxman, T. E., Schneider, L. S., Arean, P. A., Alexopoulos, G. S. et al. (2002). Evidence-based practices in geriatric mental health care. *Psychiatric Services, 53*(11), 1419-1431.

Bartels, S. J., Haley, W. E., & Dums, A. R. (2002). "Implementing Evidence-Based Practices in Geriatric Mental Health." *Generations* (Spring 2002): 90-95.

Bernard-Opitz, V., Sriram, N., & Nakhoda-Sapuan, S. (2001). Enhancing social problem solving in children with autism and normal children through computer-assisted instruction. *Journal of Autism & Developmental Disorders, 34*(4), 377-384.

Bodenheimer, T., Wagner, E. H., & Grumbach, K. (2002). "Improving primary care for patients with chronic illness: The chronic care model, part 2." *Journal of the American Medical Association* 288(15): 1909-1914.

Botelho, R. J., & Skinner, H. (1995). Motivating Change in Health Behavior. *Primary Care, 22*(4), 565-589.

Burns, R., Nichols, L. O., Martindale-Adams, J., & Graney, M. J. (2000). Interdisciplinary geriatric primary care evaluation and management: Two-year outcomes. *Journal of the American Geriatrics Society, 48*(1), 8-13.

Catalan, J., Gath, D. H. et al. (1991). "Evaluation of a brief psychological treatment for emotional disorders in primary care." *Psychological Medicine* 21: 1013-1018.

Claiborne, N., & Vandenburgh, H. (2002). Social workers' role in disease management. *Health and Social Work, 26*(4), 217-224.

Cochrane, A. L. (1972). *Effectiveness and efficiency. Random reflections on health services.* London: Nuffield Provincial Hospitals Trust.

Cook, S., Herold, K., Edidin, D., & Briars, R. (2002). Increasing problem solving in adolescents with type 1 diabetes: The choices diabetes program. *Diabetes Education, 28*(1), 115-124.

Coons, S. J., Rao, S., Keininger, D. L., & Hays, R. D. (2000). A comparative review of generic quality-of-life instruments. *Pharmacoeconomics, 17*(1), 13-35.

Dowrick, C., Dunn, G. et al. (2000). "Problem solving treatment and group psychoeducation for depression: Multicentre randomized controlled trial." *British Medical Journal* 321: 1-6.

Drake, R. E., Goldman, H. H., Leff, H. S., Lehman, A. F., Dixon, L., Mueser, K. T. et al. (2001). Implementing evidence-based practices in routine mental health service settings. *Psychiatric Services, 52*(2), 179-182.

D'Zurilla, T., & Nezu, A. (1987). The Heppner and Krauskopf approach: A model of personal problem solving or social skills? *The Counseling Psychologist, 15*, 463-470.

Enguidanos, S., Davis, C., & Katz, L. (2003). "Shifting the paradigm in geriatric care management: Moving from the medical model to patient centered care." *The Journal of Health Care Social Work: A Quarterly Journal Adopted by the Society for Social Work Leadership in Health Care* 41(1): 1-26.

Flaherty, J., Morley, J., Murphy, D., & Wasserman, M. (2002). The development of outpatient clinical glidepaths. *Journal of the American Geriatrics Society, 50*(11), 1886-1901.

Gambrill, E. (2001). Social Work: Authority-Based Profession. *Research on Social Work Practice, 11*(2), 166-175.

Grant, J. S., Elliott, T. R., Giger Newman, J., & Bartolucci, A. A., (2001). "Social problem-solving telephone partnerships with family caregivers of persons with stroke." *International Journal of Rehabiliation Research* 24: 181-189.

Hegel, M. T. & Arean, P. (2003). Problem-Solving Treatment of Depression in Primary Care: A Treatment Manual, Hartford Foundation:1-133.

Kane, R. A., Kane, R. L., & Ladd, R. (1998). *The heart of long-term care.* New York: Oxford University Press.

Katz, J. N., Larson, M. G., Phillips, C. B., Fossel, A. H., & Liang, M. H. (1992). Comparative measurement sensitivity of short and longer health status instruments. *Medical Care, 30*(10), 917-925.

Kerridge, I., Lowe, M., & Henry, D. (1998). Ethics and evidence based medicine. *British Medical Journal, 316*, 1151-1153.

Kunik, M. E., Braun, U., Stanley, M. A., Wristers, K., Molinari, V., Stoebner, D. et al. (2001). One session cognitive behavioral therapy for elderly patients with chronic obstructive pulmonary disease. *Psychological Medicine, 31*, 717-723.

Lawrence, W. F., & Fleishman, J. A. (2004). Predicting EuroQoL EQ-5D preference scores from the SF-12 health survey in a nationally representative sample. *Medical Decision Making, 24*(2), 160-169.

Liberman, R., Eckman, T., & Marder, S. (2001). Training in social problem solving among persons with schizophrenia. *Psychiatric Services, 52*(1), 31-33.

Lisansky, D., & Clough, D. H. (1996). A cognitive-behavioral self-help educational program for patients with COPD. *Psychotherapy and Psychosomatics, 65*, 97-101.

Lorig, K. R. (1993). Self-Management of Chronic Illness: A Model for the Future. *Generations* (Fall 1993), 11-14.

Lorig, K. R., & Laurin, J. (1985). Some notions about assumptions underlying health education. *Health Education Quarterly, 12*(3), 231-243.

Medalia, A., Revheim, N., & Casey, M. (2001). The remediation of problem-solving skills in schizophrenia. *Schizophrenia Bulletin, 27*(2), 259-267.

Miller, W. R. (1996). Motivation Interviewing: Research, Practice, and Puzzles. *Addictive Behaviors, 21*(6), 835-842.

Morrow-Howell, N., Proctor, E. K., & Dore, P. (1998). Post-acute services to older patients with heart disease. *Journal of Applied Gerontology, 17*(2), 150-171.

Mynors-Wallis, L. M., Gath, D. H. et al. (2000). "Randomised controlled trial of problem solving treatment, antidepressant medication, and combined treatment for major depression in primary care." *British Medical Journal* 320: 26-30.

Nikolaus, T., Specht-Leible, N., Bach, M., Oster, P., & Schlierf, G. (1999). A randomized trial of comprehensive geriatric assessment and home intervention in the care of hospitalized patients. *Age and Ageing, 28*, 543-550.

Oishi, S., Shoai, R., Katon, W., Callahan, C. M., Unutzer, J., & IMPACT. (2003). Impacting late life depression: Integrating a depression intervention into primary care. *Psychiatric Quarterly, 74*(1), 75-89.

Oxman, T., & Dietrich, A. (2002). The key role of primary care physicians in mental health care for elders. *Generations*, Spring 2002.

Perlman, H. H. (1957). *Social casework: A problem-solving process* (17 ed.). Chicago: The University of Chicago Press.

Pfeiffer, E. (1975). A short portable mental status questionnaire for the assessment of organic brain deficit in elderly patients. *Journal of the American Geriatrics Society, 23*(10), 433-441.

Rizzo, V., & Rowe, J. (2003). Studies of the efficacy of social work services in aging with a focus on cost outcomes: Preliminary key points and information. *draft paper*.

Rosen, A., Proctor, E., & Staudt, M. (1999). Social work research and the quest for effective practice. *Social Work Research, 23*(1), 4-14.

Rubin, C. D., MD, Sizemore, M. T., PhD., Loftis, P. A., MS, RN, Adams-Huet, B., & Anderson, R. J. (1992). The effect of geriatric evaluation and management on Medicare reimbursement in a large public hospital: A randomized clinical trial. *Journal of the American Geriatrics Society, 40*, 989-995.

Rychetnik, L., Hawe, P., Waters, E., Barratt, A., & Frommer, M. (2004). A glossary for evidence based public health. *Journal of Epidemiology and Community Health, 58*, 538-545.

Sackett, D., Rosenberg, W., Muir Gray, J., Haynes, B., & Richardson, W. S. (1996). Evidence based medicine: What it is and what it isn't. *British Medical Journal, 312*, 71-72.

Sahler, O., Varni, J., Fairclough, D., Butler, R., Noll, R., Dolgin, M. et al. (2002). Problem-solving skills training for mothers of children with newly diagnosed cancer: A randomized trial. *Journal of Developmental and Behavioral Pediatrics, 23*(2), 77-86.

Sapin, C., Fantino, B., Nowicki, M.-L., & Kind, P. (2004). Usefulness of EQ-5D in assessing health status in primary care patients with major depressive disorder. *Health and Quality of Life Outcomes, 2*(20).

Schilling, R. F., El-Bassel, N., Finch, J. B., Roman, R. J., & Hanson, M. (2002). Motivational Interviewing to Encourage Self-Help Participation Following Alcohol Detoxification. *Research on Social Work Practice, 12*(6), 711-730.

Schwartz, M., Lerman, C., Audrain, J., Cella, D., Rimer, B., Stefanek, M. et al. (1998). The impact of a brief problem-solving training intervention for relatives of recently diagnosed breast cancer patients. *Annals of Behavioral Medicine, 20*(1), 7-12.

Sheikh, J. I., & Yesavage, J. A. (1985). A knowledge assessment test for geriatric psychiatry. *Hospital & Community Psychiatry, 36*(11), 1160-1166.

Straus, S., & McAlister, F. (2000). Evidence-based medicine: A commentary on common criticisms. *Canadian Medical Association Journal, 163*(7), 837-841.

Teri, L., Logsdon, R. G., Uomoto, J., & McCurry, S. M. (1997). Behavior treatment of depression in dementia patients: A controlled clinical trial. *Journal of Gerontology, 52B*, 159-166.

Tickle-Degnen, L., & Bedell, G. (2003). Heterarchy and hirearchy: A critical appraisal of the "levels of evidence" as a tool for clinical decision making. *The American Journal of Occupational Therapy, 57*(2), 234-237.

Unutzer, J. (2002). Diagnosis and treatment of older adults with depression in primary care. *Biological Psychiatry, 52*, 285-292.

Unutzer, J., Katon, W., Sullivan, M., & Miranda, J. (1999). Treating depressed older adults in primary care: Narrowing the gap between efficacy and effectiveness. *The Milbank Quarterly, 77*(2), 225-256.

Wagner, E. H., Austin, B. T., Davis, C., Hindmarsh, M., Schaefer, J., & Bonomi, A. E. (2001). Improving chronic illness care: Translating evidence into action; interventions that encourage people to acquire self-management skills are essential to chronic illness care. *Health Affairs.*

Wagner, E. H., Austin, B. T., & Von Korff, M. (1996). Improving outcomes in chronic illness. *Managed Care Quarterly, 4*(2), 12-25.

Ware, J. E. J., Kosinski, M., & Keller, S. (1996). A 12-item short-form health survey: Construction of scales and preliminary tests of reliability and validity. *Medical Care, 34*(3), 220-233.

Ware, J. J., & Sherbourne, C. D. (1992). The MOS 36-item short-form health survey (SF-36). I. Conceptual framework and item selection. *Medical Care, 30*, 473-483.

West, R. (2000). Editorial: Evidence based medicine overviews, bulletins, guidelines, and the new consensus. *PMJ Online, 76*, 383-389.

Williams, J. W., J. Barrett et al. (2000). Treatment of Dysthymia and Minor Depression in Primary Care: A Randomized Controlled Trial in Older Adults. *Journal of the American Medical Association, 284*(12): 1519-1526.

Williams, M. E., MD, Williams, T. F., MD, Zimmer, J. G., MD, Hall, W. J., PhD, & Podgorski, C. A., MS. (1987). How does the team approach to outpatient geriatric evaluation compare with traditional care: A report of a randomized controlled trial. *Journal of the American Geriatrics Society, 35*(12), 1071-1078.

Zanis, D., Coviello, D., Alterman, A., & Appling, S. (2001). A community-based trial of vocational problem-solving to increase employment among methadone patients. *Journal of Substance Abuse Treatment, 21*, 19-26.

Depression Care for the Elderly: Reducing Barriers to Evidence-Based Practice

Kathleen Ell, DSW

SUMMARY. This paper provides an overview of five key bodies of evidence identifying: (1) *Characteristics of depression among older adults*–its prevalence, risk factors and illness course, and impact on functional status, mortality, use of health services, and health care costs; (2) *Effective Interventions*, including pharmacologic, psychotherapies, care management, and combined intervention models; (3) *Known Barriers to depression care* including patient, provider and service system barriers; (4) *Effective Organizational and Educational Strategies* to reduce barriers to depression care; and (5) *Key Factors in Translating Research into Practice*. There is strong empirical support for implementing strategies to improve depression care for older adults. *[Article copies available for a fee from The Haworth Document Delivery Service: 1-800-HAWORTH. E-mail address: <docdelivery@haworthpress.com> Website: <http://www.HaworthPress.com> © 2006 by The Haworth Press, Inc. All rights reserved.]*

Address correspondence to: Kathleen Ell, DSW, School of Social Work, MRF 102R (MC 0411), University of Southern California, Los Angeles, CA 90089-0411 (E-mail: ell@usc.edu).

The work on this manuscript was supported, in part, by NIMH grant 5 R24 MH61700-02 (Dr. Ell, PI).

[Haworth co-indexing entry note]: "Depression Care for the Elderly: Reducing Barriers to Evidence-Based Practice." Ell, Kathleen. Co-published simultaneously in *Home Health Care Services Quarterly* (The Haworth Press, Inc.) Vol. 25, No. 1/2, 2006, pp. 115-148; and: *Evidence-Based Interventions for Community Dwelling Older Adults* (ed: Susan M. Enguídanos) The Haworth Press, Inc., 2006, pp. 115-148. Single or multiple copies of this article are available for a fee from The Haworth Document Delivery Service [1-800-HAWORTH, 9:00 a.m. - 5:00 p.m. (EST). E-mail address: docdelivery@haworthpress.com].

KEYWORDS. Major depression, elderly, evidence-based practice, primary care, home health care, barriers to depression care, collaborative depression care

INTRODUCTION

Clinical depression is prevalent among older adults and negatively affects functional status, quality of life and mortality, while increasing health care costs and taking a toll on family caregivers. Unfortunately, despite the availability of effective treatments for depressed elders, the majority remain untreated or undertreated–attributable to well-documented patient, health provider, service system, and social-structural barriers to ensuring that optimal care and services are accessible to elders (Charney, Reynolds, Lewis, Lebowitz, Sunderland, Alexopoulos et al., 2003; Unützer, 2002).

Defining evidence-based practice solely as "evidence-based treatment" fails to adequately address known barriers to depression care. A more useful and comprehensive definition "empirically supported practice" includes evidence on: patient care seeking and adherence behavior; provider knowledge, clinical decision making and care management skills; health care system design or redesign; and organizational incentives and resources that lead to the implementation of evidence based practice and program guidelines, and empirically derived quality monitoring indicators. This paper provides an overview of five key bodies of evidence identifying: (1) *Characteristics of depression among older adults*–its prevalence, risk factors and illness course, and impact on functional status, mortality, use of health services, and health care costs; (2) *Effective Interventions*, including pharmacologic, psychotherapies, care management, and combined intervention models; (3) *Known Barriers to depression care* including patient, provider and service system barriers; (4) *Effective Organizational and Educational Strategies* to Reduce Barriers to depression care; and (5) *Key Factors in Translating Research into Practice*.

CHARACTERISTICS OF LATE-LIFE DEPRESSION

In community-dwelling older adults, the prevalence of major depression is estimated to be 1%-4% (Mojtabai & Olfson, 2004; Steffens, Skoog,

Norton, Hart, Tschanz, Plassman et al., 2000) and of subsyndromal depression 15 to 30% (Beekman, Deeg, Braam, Smit & VanTilburg, 1997; Lavretsky & Kunar, 2002; Lebowitz, Pearson, Schneider, Reynolds, Alexopoulos, Bruce et al., 1997; Montgomery et al., 2000). The latter include elderly with depressive syndromes such as dysthymia, bereavement, adjustment disorder with depressed mood and minor depression along a spectrum of illness severity that results in significant functional morbidity (Flint, 2002; Lyness, 2004; Unützer, 2002). Prevalence of major or clinically significant depression among medically ill elderly ranges from 10 to 43% (Charney et al., 2003). Depression is the most common late life mental disorder to present in community based primary care. About 1 in 10 primary care patients has major depression, with increasing depression prevalence in home health care (10-26%) (Bruce et al., 1998; Banerjee & McDonald, 1996; Ell et al., 2004; Ell & Enguidanos, 2004), and nursing homes (12-30%) (Hendrie, Callahan, Levitt, Hui, Musick, Austrom et al., 1995; Jongenelis, Pot, Eises, Beekman, Kluiter & Ribbe, 2004; Unützer, Patrick, Simon, Grembowski, Walker, Rutter et al., 1997). Rates of depression in older adults are higher among women (Blazer, Burchett, Service & George, 1991). Prevalence rates are similar between African-American and White elderly (Bazargan & Hamm-Baugh, 1995), and may be higher among less acculturated Hispanics (González, Haan & Hinton, 2001).

Among the elderly, physical illness and disability are major risk factors for depression (Jorm, 1998; Koenig et al., 1998; Roberts et al., 1997) as are cognitive deficits, declining functional status, social network losses and low social support, and negative life events (Bruce, 2002; Devanand, Kim, Paykina & Sackeim, 2002; Krasij, Arensman, Spinhover, 2002; Mojtabai & Olfson, 2004; Pennix, Guralnik, Ferrucci, Simonsick, Deeg, D., & Wallace, 1998; Ranga, George, Peiper, Jiang, Arias, Look et al., 1998; West et al., 1998). Comorbidity of depression with other medical diseases in the elderly is common (Ranga, Krishnan, Delong, Kraemer, Carney, Spiegel et al., 2002) and medical illness increases the risk of suicide in the elderly (Juurlink, Hermann, Szalai, Kopp & Redelmeier, 2004; Suominen, Henriksson, Isometsa, Conwell, Heila & Lonnqvist, 2003).

Higher rates of disability, impaired quality of life and mortality are found among depressed elders (Alexopoulos, Vrontou, Kakuma, Meyers, Young, Klausner & Clarkin, 1996; Cronin-Stubbs, deLeon, Beckett, Field, Glynn & Evans, 2000; Black, Markides & Ray, 2003; Doraiswamy, Khan, Donahue & Richard, 2002; de Jonge, Ormel, Slaets, Gertrudis, Kempen, Ranchor et al., 2004; Lavretsky, Bastani, Gould, Huang, Llorente Maxwell et al., 2002; Stein & Barrett-Connor,

2002; Pulska, Pahkala, Laippala & Kivela, 1998; Unützer, Patrick, Marmon, Simon & Katon, 2002). The likely multiple pathways that underly the effect of depression on mortality are only beginning to be understood (Alexopoulos & Chester, 1992; Covinsky, Fortinsky, Palmer, Kresevic & Landefeld, 1997; Ariyo, Haan, Tangen, Rutledge, Cushman, Dobs et al., 2002; Katz, 1996; Mehta, Yaffe, Langa, Sands, Whooley, & Covinsky, 2003; Schulz, Drayer & Rollman, 2002).

For many elderly patients, major depression has a chronic course–persistent, intermittent, and/or recurrent (Beekman et al., 2002; Cole, 1999; Lyness, Caine, King, Conwell, Duberstein, Cox, 2002; Raue et al., 2003; Mueller et al., 2004; Unutzer et al., 1997; 1999). Recent studies of treatment response and illness course among elderly patients find that clinical factors such as history, duration, and severity of depression, comorbid physical illness and disability, and antidepressant treatment as well as psychosocial factors, such as basic and instrumental social support predict depression treatment response, illness course, functional decline and even mortality (Bosworth, McQuoid, George & Steffens, 2002; Hays, Steffens, Flint, Bosworth & George, 2001; Geerlings, Beekman, Deeg, Twisk & Vantilburg, 2002). In the medically ill, improvement or lack of improvement in depression and disability following hospitalization are frequently closed related (Koenig & George, 1998). Depression recovery may be slower in the elderly (Thomas, Mulsant, Solano, Black, Bensai, Flynn et al., 2002).

Late onset, unipolar depression is particularly characteristic of elderly suicides (Conwell et al., 1996; Dennis & Lindesay, 1995; Henriksson, Marttunen, Isometsä, Heikkinen, Aro, Kuoppasalmi et al., 1995). For the most part, older suicide victims have had late onset undetected or untreated depressions, although typically they have had contact with their primary care provider prior to their death (Suominen et al., 2004). And depression may influence end-of-life decision-making as in the case of depressed elderly found to initially decline cardiopulmonary resuscitation, but accept it after recovery from depression (Eggar, Spencer, Anderson & Hiller, 2002).

Not surprising, given its prevalence in medically ill elderly, depression is also associated with increased health service use (Beekman, Deeg, Braam, Smit, & VanTilburg, 1997; Koenig & Kutchibhatla, 1999) and medical costs (Katon, Lin, Russo & Unützer, 2003). Gender differences in depression, service utilization and treatment cost among Medicare elderly raise important questions. In a 5% random sample of 35,673 Medicare beneficiaries, females had a significantly higher incidence of major and other depression and higher outpatient and mental health care costs; whereas total health care costs were higher for men (Burns, Cain, & Husaini, 2001). And depression in medically ill elders can result in increased burden on family caregivers (Langa, Valenstein, Fendrick, Kabeto, & Vijan Langa, 2004; Sewitch, McCusker, Dendukuri & Yaffe, 2004).

In summary, the evidence on characteristics of late-life depression supports the need to address depression in the elderly. Routine patient education, screening, and evaluation in older adults with known risk factors are particularly recommended. For example, efforts to improve treatment of depression in primary care have led to lowered suicide rates (Rutz, von Knorring & Wålinder, 1989; Rihmer, Rutz, & Pihlgren, 1995), resulting in recommendations that late-life suicide prevention focus on adequate recognition and treatment of depression (Conwell & Duberstein, 1995; Lish, Zimmerman, Farber, Lush, Kuzma, M.A., & Plescia, 1996; Rihmer, 1996).

EFFECTIVE PHARMACOLOGICAL AND PSYCHOTHERAPEUTIC TREATMENT IN THE ELDERLY

Pharmacologic Treatment

Treatment studies document the safety and efficacy of anti-depressant treatment among older adults (Bump, Mulsant, Pollock, Mazumdar, Begley, Dew & Reynolds, 2001; das Gupta, 1998; Salzman, Wong & Wright, 2002), with SSRI's being generally less toxic than older medications (Charney et al., 2003; Sheikh, Cassidy, Doraiswamy, Salomon, Hornig, Holland, Mandel, Clary & Burt et al., 2004). Between 60-80% of patients will respond to medications if prescribed according to recommended guidelines, although full therapeutic benefit may take 8-12 weeks and only about half of patients respond to the first medication prescribed (Sable, Dunn & Zisook, 2002). Response time may be longer among suicidal, more severely depressed and patients with comorbid anxiety (Szanto, Mulsant, Houck, Dew & Reynolds, 2003; Whyte, Dew, Gildengers, Lenze, Bharucha, Mulsant et al., 2004). Therapy should be continued for at least 6 months, while patients at risk for relapse frequently require therapy for up to 2 years or indefinitely (Sable et al., 2002). There is some evidence that antidepressants are effective for frail elders, for patients with dysthymia and more severely impaired elders with minor depression (Strein et al., 2000; Williams, Barrett, Oxman, Frank, Katon, Sullivan et al., 2000). However, questions remain about the effectiveness of antidepressants for the older adults because few trials have been conducted in the elderly, only a relatively small number of studies address elderly with comorbid conditions, and there is evidence of a significant placebo response rate and a significant number of elders who do not respond or have residual depressive symptoms (Taylor & Doraiswany, 2004).

To reduce inappropriate medication prescribing (Goulding, 2004), pharmacologic guidelines are available to assist primary care physicians in medication management (Dunner, 2003; Serby & You, 2003), however, patients with comorbid illness and accompanying complications and drug-drug interactions may require adapting general guidelines (Sable et al., 2002). For example, for older adults with pain symptoms, combining antidepressant and pain pharmacotherapy may be indicated (Rao & Cohen, 2004; Unützer, Ferrell, Lin & Marmon, 2004). Poor patient adherence, as well as social factors can negatively affect treatment response (Sable et al., 2002). To address adherence and social problems that negatively affect treatment response, patient education and sometimes brief counseling is required (Sable et al., 2002).

Structured Psychosocial Therapies

There is growing consensus that structured psychotherapy, alone or combined with antidepressant treatment, is effective for older adults with depression (Areán et al., 2001; Areán & Cook, 2002; Areán et al., 1993; Gum & Areán, 2004; Leibowitz et al., 1997; Unützer et al., 1999). Under some circumstances it is the treatment of choice (i.e., when preferred by individual patients, when pharmacologic treatments are contraindicated, and for elders coping with low social support or environmental stressors), or for maintenance after discontinuation of antidepressant medication (Reynolds et al., 1999). Clinical benefits from psychotherapy should be evident within 6-8 weeks and are frequently maintained among the elderly for up to a year. Medications should be considered for patients who fail to improve by that time and for those who do not have a full remission after 12 weeks of psychotherapy. Structured psychosocial therapies are as effective as antidepressants for moderate depression and may be more effective in reducing recurrence.

Manualized cognitive behavioral therapies have been shown to be effective in depressed older adults, including elders with comorbid physical illness and disability, cognitive impairment, or comorbid anxiety (Areán & Cook, 2002; Kunik, Braun, Stanley, Wristers, Molinari, Stoebner et al., 2001; Lenze, 2003; Thompson, Coon, Gallagher-Thompson, Sommer &

Koin, 2001). Cognitive-Behavioral Therapy (CBT) challenges pessimistic or self-critical thoughts, emphasizing rewarding activities and decreasing behavior that reinforces depression. Alernative modes of delivery of CBT have been explored, including group CBT and telephone or computer self-help formats (Proudfoot, Goldberg, Mann, Everitt, Marks & Gray, 2003). Problem-Solving Treatment (PST) teaches patients to address current life problems by identifying smaller elements of larger problems and specific steps toward solving these. PST, adapted for primary care (PST-PC) in the multi-site IMPACT study (Haverkamp, Areán, Hegel & Unützer, 2003; Kindy, 2003) was found to significantly reduce depressive symptoms among older primary care patients with major depression or dysthymia, including among African-American and Hispanic patients (Unützer et al., 2002) and among elders with major depression and executive dysfunction (Alexopoulos, Raire & Areán, 2003). PST has also been adapted for older adult home care patients in an ongoing study (Ell & Enguidanos, 2004) and for low-income Latinos with cancer (Dwight-Johnson, Ell & Lee, 2005). CBT has been adapted for elderly Chinese Americans (Dai, Zhang, Yamamoto, Ao, Belin, Cheung et al., 1999).

Interpersonal Therapy (IPT) combines elements of psychodynamic-oriented and cognitive therapies to address interpersonal difficulties, role transitions, and unresolved grief. The majority of studies with older adults have combined IPT with medication or pill-placebo (Areán & Cook, 2002). Combining IPT with antidepressant medication is effective in reducing symptoms in older adults, may prevent relapse and is effective as a maintenance treatment for more severely depressed older adults (Miller, Cornes, Frank, Ehrenpreis, Silberman, Schlernitzaues et al., 2001; Miller, Frank, Cornes, Houck & Reynolds, 2003; Reynolds, Dew, Frank, Begley, Miller, Cornes et al., 1998; Reynolds, Frank, Perel, Imber, Cornes, Miller et al., 1999; Taylor, Reynolds, Cornes, Miller, Stack, Begley et al., 1999; Scocco & Frank, 2002).

BARRIERS TO DEPRESSION CARE FOR THE ELDERLY

Undetected and Inadequately Treated

Although recent evidence indicates that antidepressant use is increasing among Medicare patients (Crystal, Sambamoorthi, Walkup & Akincigil, 2003; Sambamoorthi, Olfson, Walkup & Crystal, 2003), the majority of depressed elderly do not receive antidepressant treatment (Charney et al.,

2003; Luber, Meyers & Williams-Russo, Hollenberg, DiDomenico, Charlson, Alexopoulos, 2001; Unützer et al., 2000). Few depressed older medical patients receive antidepressants in the hospital and even fewer are treated after discharge (Engberg, Sereika, Weber, Engberg, McDowell & Reynolds, 2001; Koenig et al., 1997) or in home health care (Bruce, McAvay, Raue, Brown, Meyers, Keohane et al., 2002). Older suicide victims have had late onset depressions that are not detected or treated, although typically they have had contact with their primary care provider prior to their death (Pfaff & Almeida, 2004). Elderly persons are also less likely to receive an adequate course of psychotherapy compared to younger adults (Harman, Edlund & Fortney, 2004). Older men, patients who prefer counseling or psychotherapy, and racial/ethnic minority elders are less likely to receive any depression care (Brown et al., 1995; Green-Hennessy & Hennessy, 1999; Areán & Unützer, 2003; Sclar, Robinson, Skaer et al., 1999; Unützer, Katon, Callahan, Williams, Hunkeler, Harpole et al., 2003; Virnig, Huang, Lurie, Musgrave, McBean & Dowd, 2004). Poor elderly with Medicaid are also disadvantaged (Crystal et al., 2003; Melfi, Crogan & Hanna, 1999; 2000). Efforts to increase access to care and to improve the quality of depression care for older adults will need to address important patient, provider, and health system barriers to care (see Figure 1).

Patient Barriers

Patient barriers to depression care influence detection and treatment processes. For example, older patients are less likely to voluntarily report depressive symptoms, may view depression as a moral weakness or character flaw, not an illness, and may be more likely to ascribe symptoms of depression to a physical illness (Heithoff, 1995; Knauper & Wittchen, 1994; Lyness, Cox, Curry, Conwell, King & Caine, 1995). Perceived stigma of depression has been associated with treatment discontinuation among older patients and treatment non-adherence (Sirey, Bruce, Alexopoulos, Perlick, Friedman & Meyers, 2001; Sirey, Bruce, Alexopoulos, Perlick, Raue, Friedman et al., 2001). Nonadherence to treatment among the elderly is common (Maidment, Livingston & Katona, 2002; Salzman, 1995; Wetherell & Unützer, 2003), perhaps due in part to elders' doubts that medication is helpful (Prabhakaran & Butler, 2002). Depressed older adults are less likely to use specialty mental health care, preferring to use the general health care system (Bartels, Coakley, Zubritsky, Ware, Miles, Areán et al., 2004) and may be reluctant to attend group psychotherapy, but more willing to attend

FIGURE 1. Evidence-Based Barriers to Depression Care for Older Adults

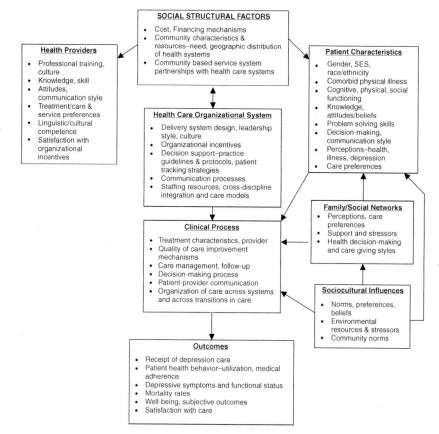

psychoeducational therapy formats (Areán, Alvidrez, Barrera, Robinson & Hicks, 2002).

Culturally based preferences for depression care can become a barrier to care if the preferred mode of care is not available (Cooper-Patrick et al., 1997). Personal culturally based explanations for depression symptoms may influence symptom expression and patient-provider communication (Gallo et al., 1998; Lin et al., 1995; Marwaha & Livingston, 2002; Melfi et al., 1999; Mills, Alea & Cheong, 2004). Patient perceptions of bias and cultural competence in health care, family perceptions, and practical barriers such as cost and transportation to therapy may impede receipt of care (Johnson, Saha, Arbelaez, Beach & Cooper, 2004).

Provider Barriers

The majority of older adults receive antidepressants from primary care physicians (Harman, Crystal, Walkup & Olfson, 2003). Physician attitudes and experiences may affect depression treatment more than knowledge (Areán, Alvidrez, Feldman, Tong & Shermer, 2003; Poutanen, 1996; Williams, Rost, Dietrich, Ciotti, Zyzanski & Cornell, 1999). Physicians may miss depression because they assume it is a "natural" consequence of aging and associated physical illness, or fail to initiate treatment due to doubts about the efficacy of treatment (Alvidrez & Areán, 2002). Primary care physicians may be more likely to detect depression in older women compared to men, because they are more likely to report affective symptoms and crying spells (Allen-Burge et al., 1994; Brown et al., 1995).

Not surprising, physical problems compete with depression for physician attention, thus potentially decreasing the odds that the elderly will receive guideline level pharmacological or psychotherapy treatment (Bartels, Dums, Oxman, Schneider, Areán, Alexopoulos, & Jeste, 2002; Moser, 2002). For example, elderly hospitalized patients who remained depressed and physically disabled following hospitalization do not see mental health specialists any more frequently than elderly without depression or physical impairment (Koenig & Kuchibhatla, 1999). Physicians may fail to distinguish severity levels of depression or depression from social problems. As a result, they may inadequately manage depression, emphasize possible organic pathology, fail to elicit mood or cognitive symptoms, underestimate symptoms in the most severely depressed, including patients at risk of suicide (Fischer, Wei, Solberg, Rush & Heinrich, 2003; Volkers, Nuyen, Verhaak & Schellevis, 2004), and may be less willing to treat suicidal ideation (Uncapher & Areán, 2000). Physicians also report that guidelines are insufficiently flexible for the variety of patients seen in primary care (Smith, Walker & Gilhooly, 2004).

Recent studies find that home health care nurses may also fail to identify late-life depression (Bruce et al., 2002; Bruno & Ahrens, 2003; Raue, Brown & Bruce, 2002; Brown, McAvay, Raue, Moses & Bruce, 2003; Brown, Bruce, McAvay, Raue & Lachs et al., 2004). Sole reliance on home care nurse clinical judgment is reported to be inadequate when compared to the use of structured screening tools (Ell et al., 2004; Preville, Cote, Boyer, & Hebert, 2004). Nurses may lack specific training in depression and may be uncomfortable with assessing depression (Larson, Chernoff & Sweet-Holp, 2004; McDonald, Passik, Dugan, Rosenfeld & Theobald et al., 1999; Williams & Payne, 2003). Lack of educational support and ease of access to mental health specialists are found to be principal barriers that accounted for nurses' reluctance to uncover mental health problems (Nolan, Murray & Dallender, 1999).

Health System Barriers

Organizational system barriers may limit implementation of depression guidelines or quality of care improvements. These include lack of coordination and collaboration between providers in primary care, long-term care and specialty mental health providers and shortages of nursing and social service professionals who have training and expertise in geriatric mental health (Bartels et al., 2002). Economic barriers can interact with organizational barriers. Inadequate or discriminatory financing of mental health services for older adults may defer care (Bartels et al., 2002). Capitated payment systems that effectively create incentives to provide fewer services or lack of mechanisms to pay for depression care provided by nurses or social workers are examples (Frank, Huskamp & Pincus, 2003). Inadequate drug coverage and the high cost of drugs may deter elders using antidepressants or taking less than recommended doses to reduce costs (Ganguli, 2003; Goldman, Joyce, Escarce, Pace, Solomon et al., 2004).

EFFECTIVE STRATEGIES TO IMPROVE THE DELIVERY OF DEPRESSION CARE FOR THE ELDERLY

Depression care quality improvement strategies have been shown to be effective in reducing barriers to depression care (Badamgarav, Weingarten, Henning, Knight, Hasselblad, Gano et al., 2003; Gilbody et al., 2003; Mulsant, Whyte, Lenze, Lotrich, Karp, Pollock et al., 2003)–including among racial/ethnic minorities (Wells, Sherbourne, Schoenbaum, Ettner, Duan, Miranda et al., 2004). Organizational and educational strategies have been most frequently studied. Modest or mixed results stem from provider education and usually are most effective when combined with more complex interventions that bring additional resources into the health care system (Cherry, Vickrey, Schwankovsky, Heck, Plauchm & Yep, 2004; Gilbody, Whitty, Grimshaw & Thomas, 2003). Aimed at reducing patient barriers to care, patient and sometimes family education seeking their active engagement in depression care management is particularly promising. Organizational strategies (Reuben, 2002) generally include multifaceted quality improvement disease management interventions that change the way depression care is delivered, such as the implementation of routine depression screening, systematic application of evidence-based practice guidelines, clinical decision-making protocols and algorithms, follow-up through remission and maintenance, enhanced roles of nurses or social workers as depression care managers as well as integration between primary care and mental health specialists or service systems.

Effective Screening and Diagnostic Tools and Practice Guidelines

Tools to facilitate routine screening or physician assessment are designed to reduce failure to detect depression. In recent years, the 9-item Patient Health Questionnaire (PHQ-9) (Kroenke, Spitzer & Williams, 2001) has emerged as one of the most reliable depression screening tools in primary care with a demonstrated ability to identify clinically important depression, to make accurate diagnoses of major depression (Kroenke & Spitzer, 2002), to track severity of depression over time (Löwe et al., 2004) and to monitor patient response to therapy (Löwe, Unützer, Callahan, Perkins & Kroenke, 2004). The instrument is valid and reliable (Spitzer, Kroenke & Williams, 1999), has specific diagnostic criteria and clinically significant cutoff scores (Kroenke et al., 2001), and has been used with older adults in the IMPACT primary care study where it was found to be sensitive to change in symptom severity when compared with a longer standardized depression severity measure (Löwe et al., 2004a), and can be administered in-person or via telephone (Simon, Ludman, Tutty, Operskalski & von Korff, 2004). Other symptom screening tools are available, as are guidelines for brief, but reliable clinical examination by primary care physicians (Williams, Noel, Cordes, Ramirez & Pignone, 2002). Routine screening of patients with known risk factors is particularly likely to improve care (Schulberg, Bruce, Lee, Williams & Dietrich, 2004).

To improve optimal treatment, there are well-established clinical practice guidelines, consensus statements, and decision-making algorithms for managing depression in older adults (Kurlowicz, 2003; Lebowitz et al., 1997; Sable et al., 2002; Sommer, Fenn, Pompei, DeBattista, Lembke, Wang & Flores, 2003; Unützer et al., 2002). Clinical guidelines are available on professional and organizational websites and address depression care by primary care physicians, nurses, and community based clinics (*www.depression-primarycare.org/clinicians/*; *www.guidelines.gov/summary/summary.aspx?doc_id=3512&nbr=738&string= depression*), including important adaptations for home health care practices (Peterson, 2004).

Effective Health System-Focused Models of Care

Health system-focused depression care models bring new resources into the general health sector or into community agencies, apply clinical guideline care management, activate patient participation in their depression care, and provide patient follow-up and feedback among providers of care. Depression care models that use collaboration between primary care physicians and mental health professionals, where expertise in psychopharmacology in treating depression is provided by a psychiatrist and psychosocial interventions are provided by depression specialist nurses or social workers, are particularly promising approaches to improving depression care for the elderly. Randomized trials have shown collaborative care models to be effective in increasing the motivation of patients to cooperate with treatment, improving the primary care physician's treatment of depression, and enhancing follow-up care. While further research is needed, there is evidence that collaborative care may be cost-effective (Pyne, Rost, Zhang, Williams, Smith & Fortney, 2003; Simon, Katon, VonKorff et al., 2001; Schoenbaum et al., 2001), including for ethnic minority patients (Pirraglia, Rosen, Hermann, Olchanski & Neumann, 2004; Schoenbaum, Miranda, Sherbourne, Duan & Wells, 2004).

In the randomized study Improving Mood-Promoting Access to Collaborative Treatment (IMPACT), collaborative care using a depression care manager to support antidepressant medication treatment was effective in improving depressive symptoms and functional outcomes in adults 60 and older with major depression or dysthymia (Unützer et al., 2002). A nurse or in some cases a social worker was the designated depression clinical specialist. The depression specialist's time was primarily devoted to clinical care, including providing PST-PC, much of which was delivered by telephone (Harpole, Stechuchak, Saur, Steffens, Unützer & Oddone, 2003; Haverkamp et al., 2003).

The Prevention of Suicide in Primary Care Elderly: Collaborative Trial (PROSPECT) randomly tested collaborative care for older adults with either major depression or clinically significant minor depression. Intervention group patients received antidepressant medication or for those declining medication, the offer of brief IPT based on a clinical algorithm, and depression care management by care managers (Bruce et al., 2004). The intervention substantially reduced suicidal ideation and depression symptom severity.

The Program to Encourage Active, Rewarding Lives for Seniors (PEARLS), a community-integrated model for treating minor depression and dysthymia, tested in a randomized trial, was found to reduce depression symptoms and improve health status in medically ill, low-income, mostly homebound older adults (Ciechanowski et al., 2004). Patients were recruited through community senior service agencies by social workers who routinely screened elders during scheduled visits or telephone calls and through letters mailed by collaborating agencies to their clients or residents in affiliated public housing.

Two studies have demonstrated improved depression care for home health care patients. Flaherty and colleagues (1998) found that a multi-faceted collaborative management home care intervention for depression resulted in lower hospitalization rates (23.5%) compared to a historical control group (40.6%). A randomized controlled trial with blind follow-up six months after recruitment found that care by a psychogeriatric team home care versus usual primary care improved depressive outcomes for 58% versus 25% of people 65 and over (Banerjee et al., 1996).

The Primary Care Research in Substance Abuse and Mental Health for the Elderly (PRISM-E) randomized study compared integrated behavioral health care with enhanced referral care in primary care settings across the United States (Gallo, Zubritsky, Maxwell et al., 2004). Integrated care had mental health and substance abuse specialists within the primary care practices; the enhanced referral model included transportation, case management, and other services to engage elderly patients in treatment. Primary care clinicians strongly preferred integrated care.

Collaborative interventions also improve patient adherence and prevent relapse (Lin, VonKorff, Ludman, Rutter, Bush, Simon et al., 2003). Because depression frequently occurs with other chronic disease, adversely affecting the course of coronary heart disease, cancer, diabetes and arthritis, researchers have begun to examine whether enhancing care for depression improves depression and outcomes of these illnesses (Koike, Unützer & Wells, 2002). The collaborative care model used in the IMPACT study improved affective and functional status, but only minimally affected diabetes outcomes (Williams, Katon, Lin, Noel, Worchel, Cornell et al., 2004). Among older adults with arthritis, benefits included reduced depression, decreased pain and improved functional status and quality of life (Lin, Katon, VonKorff, Tang, Williams, Kroenke et al., 2003).

Effective Patient and Provider Educational Strategies

Patient education and activation through peer led educational group formats has been found to be effective in the ongoing management of chronic illness (Lorig & Holman, 2003; Shoor & Lorig, 2002), holding promise for similar programs in depression. Much effort has been expended trying to improve the depression care skills of primary care physicians, but with modest effect (Azocar, Cuffel, Goldman & McCarter, 2003; Callahan, 2001). Grand rounds and simply disseminating guidelines are less effective than academic detailing through brief one-on-one educational sessions (Soumerai, 1998).

Compared to other health professions, there is evidence that nurses are more likely to be willing to participate in geriatric education workshops and have high interest in mental health and dementia training (Larson, Chernoff & Sweet-Holp, 2004; Mayall, Oathamshaw, Lovell & Pusey, 2004). Thus, educational strategies aimed at increasing nurses' comfort and skill in depression assessment and care management are likely to be successful (Fazi & Wright, 2003; Ell et al., 2004; Groh & Hoes, 2003; Rosen, Mulsant, Kollar, Kastango, Mazumdar, & Fox, 2002; van Eyk, Diederikas, Kempen, Honig, van de Meer & Brenninkmeijer, 2004).

TRANSLATING RESEARCH INTO PRACTICE: RECOMMENDATIONS

Unfortunately, the availability of a strong evidence base does not ensure wide adoption of these practices in existing service systems. Despite mounting evidence that older patients tolerate and respond to treatment with antidepressants or structured psychotherapy, outcomes under real world conditions remain poor (Mulsant, Whyte, Lenze, Lotrich, Kar, Pollock & Reynolds, 2003). Improvement in late-life depression care and outcomes for a larger number of depressed elders depends on success in disseminating and implementing quality of care improvements in diverse settings. Fortunately, researchers have also begun to identify key factors in the dissemination and implementation of evidence based quality of care improvements (Bartels et al., 2002; Meresman, Hunkeler, Hargreaves, Kirsch, Robinson, Green et al., 2003; Oishi, Shoai, Katon, Callahan, Unützer et al., 2003; Pearson, Katz, Soucie, Hunkeler, Meresman, Rooney et al., 2003).

At the level of the *health system*, there must be "buy-in" for adopting a chronic care intervention from *engaged leaders and administrators* who identify the project as important and translate it into clear goals identifiable in policies, procedures, a business plan, and financial plans (ICIC, 2002c). Roles of senior management and strong clinical leaders are particularly important, including the degree to which these key people believe that the evidence responds to significant organizational or clinical needs (Bradley, Webster, Baker, Schlesinger, Inouye, Barth et al., 2004). Additional important facilitating factors are credible supportive evidence and a health care system infrastructure dedicated to translating the research into practice. Barriers are likely to emerge in relation to the extent to which changes in organizational culture are required, and the amount of coordination needed across departments or disciplines.

The Chronic Care Model (see Figure 2) provides a useful framework to guide providers who elect to provide leadership aimed at improving depression care for older adults within their system of care (www. improvingchroniccare.org/change/model/components.html). Developed by Wagner and others based on input from national experts, and extensive pilot work (ICIC, 2002a; Wagner et al., 1996a; Wagner et al., 1996b), this model recommends actions in six specific areas, including (1) the health system, (2) the community, (3) patient self-management support, (4) delivery system design, (5) provider clinical decision support, and (6) clinical information systems (see Figure 2). Intervening at the level of these components is aimed at facilitating productive interactions between patients who take an active part in their care and providers backed by resources and expertise. In turn, these interactions are designed to promote improved health status, higher satisfaction for patients and providers, and lower costs.

FIGURE 2. The Chronic Care Model

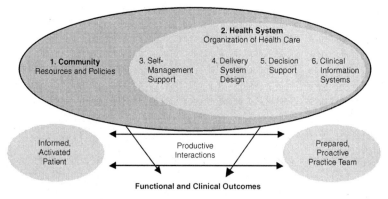

www.improvingchroniccare.org/change/model/components.html

Personnel must be provided with required resources and support to ensure change, and patients should find services convenient and affordable. Health system level changes may be essential in addressing the attitudes, social norms, and perceived barriers to treatment among providers and lower-level managers. Particularly important, the studies reviewed above emphasize the importance of integrating mental health specialists and strategies within primary care (Oxman, Dietrich & Schulberg, 2003; Sherbourne, Wells, Duan, Miranda, Unützer, Jaycox et al., 2001).

Delivery system redesign includes using planned interactions to support evidence based care (Sheeran, Brown, Nassisi & Bruce, 2004). Providers need centralized, up-to-date information and active follow-up and outreach must be incorporated into the system, with a designated staff member available for such care. Provider targeted strategies include physician education, application of practice guidelines, physician counseling skill enhancement, application of screening and diagnostic tools, and computer assisted programs to provide management feedback to physicians. Strategies, such as easy to use implementation tool kits and well-described procedures for changing practices are available (Dietrich et al., 2004; www.depression-primarycare.org; www.Annfammed.org/cgi/content/full/2/4/301/ DC1). Routine formal screening for depression in primary care is recommended by the U.S. Preventive Services Task Force (Pignone, Gaynes, Rushton, Burchell, Orleans, Mulrow et al., 2002) and tools are available as described above.

Decision support includes delivering care consistent with the scientific evidence and using proven methods to educate providers. At the level of *decision support*, treatment decisions must be based on explicit, proven guidelines that are discussed with patients (ICIC, 2002f). Providers must have ongoing training to stay up to date, and must remain in the loop when patients are referred for specialty care, through better feedback or joint consultation. These educational interventions can impact provider attitudes, social norms, and perceived barriers to care.

Similarly, *clinical information systems* provide regular audit and feedback and timely reminders for providers and patients to prompt appropriate care (Smith et al., 2004). These may be in the form of disease registries that outline recommended care for certain conditions, and check whether individuals' treatments conform to recommended guidelines (ICIC, 2002g). Outcomes are measured and reminders given for active follow-up. For providers with many competing demands, automated reminders and administrative review may ensure timely depression follow-up care.

At the level of the *community*, available resources can be identified for supporting or expanding a health system's care for chronically ill persons (ICIC, 2002b). Partnerships (such as implemented in PEARLS (Ciechanowski et al., 2004) can be formed with community agencies that provide needed educational, social, legal, or outreach services for the depressed persons, thus expanding service without duplicating efforts. There is evidence that community-based multidisciplinary geriatric mental health treatment teams are effective (Bartels, Dums, Oxman, Schneider, Areán, Alexopoulos et al., 2002; Kohn, Goldsmith & Sedgwick, 2002). In low-income communities, forming linkages among medical, mental health, social service, and community organizations is challenging because existing relationships are often fragmented, and organizations may have scarce resources, however, collaboration and shared responsibility with community agencies may reduce administrator concern about limited resources for new programs (Torrisi & McDaniel, 2003).

At the level of *self-management support*, patients and family members or caregivers should be given education and information that empowers them to take a central role in their care, so that they may work collaboratively with providers in their ongoing treatment. For depression care, patients need to be taught about available treatment options, symptom monitoring, and engaging effectively with health care providers, family, and friends. Low-income minority patients may require additional education and training in self-empowerment techniques to be active participants in their care, given their often low levels of formal education and often disenfranchised status (Dwight-Johnson et al., 2005). Self-management programs may have to address language or cultural barriers to care and allow families to play a more central role in treatment. Helping patients to communicate more effectively with providers may also help providers overcome linguistic and cultural barriers to providing good care (Johnson et al., 2004).

CONCLUSION

The research base underpinning depression care for older adults is comprehensive and encouraging. There is strong evidence of effective methods to identify and evaluate depression in older adults and strong evidence that treatment is effective in reducing depressive symptoms and improving quality of life. There is recent encouraging evidence from Medicare data that older adults (and their caregivers) may be more willing to seek and accept antidepressant treatment. Health care providers are increasingly more likely to detect and treat depression in elderly patients. Unfortunately, critical barriers remain that preclude many older adults from receiving adequate care. Foremost among these are health care system, financing and cost factors. Compelling evidence of elder need, the availability of effective treatments, and the recent evidence of effective strategies to address even some of the more intransigent health system barriers to care demand even greater commitment to and advocacy for evidence-based depression practice in a society whose population of elderly is growing (Bartels, 2003; Lyness, 2004).

REFERENCES

Alexopoulos, G.S., Raue, P., & Areán, P. (2003). Problem-solving therapy versus supportive therapy in geriatric major depression with executive dysfunction. *American Journal of Geriatric Psychiatry, 11*, 46-52.

Alexopoulos, G.S., Vrontou, C., Kakuma, T., Meyers, B.S., Young, R.C., Klausner, E., & Clarkin, J. (1996). Disability in geriatric depression. *American Journal of Psychiatry, 153*, 877-885.

Allen-Burge, R., Storandt, M., Kinscherf, D.A., & Rubin, E.H. (1994). Sex differences in the sensitivity of two self-reported depression scales in older depression inpatients. *Psychology and Aging, 9*, 443-445.

Alvidrez, J., & Areán, P.A. (2002). Physician willingness to refer older depressed patients for psychotherapy. *International Journal of Psychiatry in Medicine, 32*(1), 21-35.

Aparasu, R., Mort, J., & Brandt, H. (2003). Psychotropic medication expenditures for community-dwelling elderly persons. *Psychiatric Services, 54*(5), 739-42.

Areán, P.A., & Cook, B.L. (2002). Psychotherapy and combined psychotherapy/pharmacotherapy for late life depression. *Biological Psychiatry, 52*, 293-303.

Areán, P.A., & Unützer, J. (2003). Inequities in depression management in low-income, minority, and old-old adults: A matter of access to preferred treatments? *Journal of American Geriatrics Sociology, 51*,1808-9.

Areán, P.A., Alvidrez, J., Barrera, A., Robinson, G.S., & Hicks, S. (2002). Would older medical patients use psychological services? *Gerontologist, 42*(3), 392-8.

Areán, P.A., Alvidrez, J., Feldman, M., Tong, L., & Shermer, R. (2003). The role of provider attitudes in prescribing antidepressants to older adults: Leverage points for effective provider education. *International Journal of Psychiatry Medicine, 33*, 241-56.

Areán, P.A., Hegel, M.T., & Reynolds, C.F. (2001). Treating depression in older medical patients with psychotherapy. *Journal of Clinical Geropsychology, 7*, 93-104.

Areán, P.A., Perri, M.G., Nezu, A.M., Schein, R.L., Christopher, F., & Joseph, T.X. (1993). Comparative effectiveness of social problem-solving therapy and reminiscence therapy as treatments for depression in older adults. *Journal of Consulting and Clinical Psychology, 61*, 1003-1010.

Ariyo, A.A., Haan, M., Tangen, C.M., Rutledge, J.C., Cushman, M., Dobs, A., & Furberg, C.D. (2000). Depressive symptoms and risks of coronary heart disease and mortality in elderly Americans. Cardiovascular Health Study Collaborative Research Group. *Circulation, 102*, 1773-9.

Azocar, F., Cuffel, B., Goldman, W., & McCarter, L. (2003). The impact of evidence-based guideline dissemination for the assessment and treatment of major depression in a managed behavioral health care organization. *Journal of Behavioral Health Services & Research, 30*(1), 109-18.

Banerjee, S., & Macdonald, A.J. (1996). Mental disorder in an elderly home care population: Associations with health and social service use. *British Journal of Psychiatry, 168*, 750-756.

Banerjee, S., Shamash, K., Macdonald, A.J.D., & Mann, A.H. (1996). Randomized controlled trial of effect of intervention by a psychogeriatric team on depression in frail elderly people at home. *British Medical Journal, 13*, 1058-1061.

Bartels, S.J. (2003). Improving the system of care for older adults with mental illness in the United States: Findings and recommendations for the President's New Freedom Commission on Mental Health. *American Journal of Geriatric Psychiatry, 11*, 486-497.

Bartels, S.J., Coakley, E.H., Zubritsky, C., Ware, J.H., Miles, K.M., Areán, P.A. et al. (2004). PRISM-E Investigators. Improving access to geriatric mental health services: A randomized trial comparing treatment engagement with integrated versus enhanced referral care for depression, anxiety, and at-risk alcohol use. *American Journal of Psychiatry, 161*(8), 1455-62.

Bartels, S.J., Dums, A.R., Oxman, T.E., Schneider, L.S., Areán, P.A., Alexopoulos, G.S., & Jeste, D.V. (2002). Evidence-based practices in geriatric mental health care. *Psychiatric Services, 53*(11), 1419-31.

Bazargan, M., & Hamm-Baugh, V.P. (1995). The relationship between chronic illness and depression in a community of urban Black elderly persons. *Journal of Gerontology, 50B*, S119-S127.

Beekman, A.T., Deeg, D.J., Braam, A.W., Smit, J.H., & VanTilburg, W. (1997). Consequences of major and minor depression in later life: A study of disability, well-being and service utilization. *Psychological Medicine, 27*, 1397-1409.

Black, S.A., & Markides, K.S. (1999). Depressive symptoms and mortality in older Mexican-Americans. *Annals of Epidemiology, 9*(1), 45-52.

Blank, K., Gruman, C., & Robinson, J.T. (2004). Case-finding for depression in elderly people: Balancing ease of administration with validity in varied treatment settings. *Journal of Gerontology: Medical Sciences, 59A*, 378-384.

Blazer, D., Burchett, D., Service, C., & George, L.K. (1991). The association of age and depression among the elderly: An epidemiologic exploration. *Journal of Gerontology: Medical Science, 46*, M210-M215.

Bodenheimer, T., Lorig, K., Holman, H., & Grumbach, K. (2002). Patient self-management of chronic disease in primary care. *JAMA, 288*(19), 2469-75.

Bosworth, H.B., McQuoid, D.R., George, L.K., & Steffens, D.C. (2002). Time-to-remission from geriatric depression: Psychosocial and clinical factors. *American Journal of Geriatric Psychiatry, 10*, 551-559.

Bradley, E.H., Webster, T.R., Baker, D., Schlesinger, M., Inouye, S.K., Barth, M.C. et al. (2004). Translating research into practice: Speeding the adoption of innovative health care programs. *Issue Brief, The Commonwealth Fund. www.cmwf.org.*

Brown, E.L., Bruce, M.L., McAvay, G.J., Raue, P.J., Lachs, M.S., & Nassisi, P. (2004). Recognition of late-life depression in home care: Accuracy of the outcome and assessment Information Set. *Journal of the American Geriatrics Society, 52,* 995-999.

Brown, E.L., McAvay, G.J., Raue, P.J., Moses, S., & Bruce, M.L. (2003). Recognition of depression among elderly recipients of home care services. *Psychiatry Services, 54,* 208-213.

Bruce, M.L. (2002). Psychosocial risk factors for depressive disorders in late life. *Biol Psychiatry, 52,* 175-184.

Bruce, M.L., McAvay, G.J., Raue, P.J., Brown, E.L., Meyers, B.S., Keohane, D.J. et al. (2002). Major depression in elderly home health care patients. *American Journal of Psychiatry, 159,* 1367-1374.

Bruce, M.L., Ten Have, T.R., Reynolds, C.F. et al. (2004). Reducing suicidal ideation and depressive symptoms in depressed older primary care patients: A randomized controlled trial. *JAMA, 291,* 1081-1091.

Bruno, L., & Ahrens, J. (2003). The importance of screening for depression in home care patients. *Caring, 22,* 54-58.

Bump, G.M., Mulsant, B.H., Pollock, B.G., Mazumdar, S., Begley, A.E., Dew, M.A., & Reynolds, C.F. 3rd. (2001). Paroxetine versus nortriptyline in the continuation and maintenance treatment of depression in the elderly. *Depression & Anxiety, 13,*38-44.

Burns, M.J., Cain, V.A., & Husaini, B.A. (2001). Depression, service utilization, and treatment costs among Medicare elderly: Gender differences. *Home Health Care Services Quarterly, 19,* 35-44.

Callahan, C.M. (2001). Quality improvement research on late life depression in primary care. *Medical Care, 39,* 772-784.

Charney, D.S., Reynolds, C.F., Lewis, L., Lebowitz, B.D., Sunderland, T., Alexopoulos, G.S. et al. (2003). Depression and Bipolar Support Alliance consensus statement on the unmet needs in diagnosis and treatment of mood disorders in late life. *Archives of General Psychology, 60,* 664-72.

Cherry, D.L., Vickrey, B.G., Schwankovsky, L., Heck, E., Plauchm, M., & Yep, R. (2004). Interventions to improve quality of care: The Kaiser Permanente-Alzheimer's Association Dementia Care Project. *American Journal of Managed Care, 10*(8), 553-60.

Chu, L., Schnelle, J.F., & Osterweil, D. (2004). Prescription analgesic and antidepressant utilization and cost among elderly Medicaid beneficiaries before and after nursing home admission. *Journal of the American Medical Directors Association, 5*(2), 75-81.

Ciechanowski, P., Wagner, E., Schmaling, K., Schwartz, S., Williams, B., Diehr, P. et al. (2004). Community-integrated home-based depression treatment in older adults: A randomized controlled trial. *JAMA, 29,* 1569-1577.

Conwell, Y., & Duberstein, P.R. (1995). Prevention of late life suicide: When, where why and how. *Psychiatric Clinical Neurosciences, 49,* S79-S83.

Cooper, L.A. et al. (2003). The acceptability of treatment for depression among African-American, Hispanic, and White primary care patients. *Medical Care, 41,* 479-489.

Cooper-Patrick, L. et al. (1997). Identification of patient attitudes and preferences regarding treatment of depression. *JGIM, 12*(7), 431-438.

Cooper-Patrick, L., Powe, N.R., Jenckes, M.W., Gonzales, J.J., Levine, D.M., & Ford, D.E. (1997). Identification of patient attitudes and preferences regarding treatment of depression. *Journal of General Internal Medicine, 12,* 431-438.

Covinsky, K.E., Fortinsky, R.H., Palmer, R.M., Kresevic, D.M., & Landefeld, C.S. (1997). Relation between symptoms of depression and health status outcomes in acutely ill hospitalized older persons. *Annals of Internal Medicine, 126,* 417-425.

Croghan, T.W., Melfi, C.A., Dobrez, D.G., & Kniesner, T.J. (1999). Effect of mental health specialty care on antidepressant length of therapy. *Medical Care, 37*(4 Suppl Lilly), AS20-3.

Cronin-Stubbs, D., de Leon, C.F., Beckett, L.A., Field, T.S., Glynn, R.J., & Evans, D.A. (2000). Six-year effect of depressive symptoms on the course of physical disability in community-living older adults. *Archives of Internal Medicine, 160,* 3074-80.

Crystal, S., Sambamoorthi, U., Walkup, J.T., & Akincigil, A. (2003). Diagnosis and treatment of depression in the elderly Medicare population: Predictors, disparities, and trends. *Journal of the American Geriatric Society, 51,* 1718-1728.

Dai, Y., Zhang, S., Yamamoto, J., Ao, M., Belin, T.R., Cheung, F., & Hifumi, S.S. (1999). Cognitive behavioral therapy of minor depressive symptoms in elderly Chinese Americans: A pilot study. *Community Mental Health Journal, 35*(6), 537-42.

deJonge, P., Ormel, J., Slaets, J., Kempen, G., Ranchor, A., van Jaarsveld, C. et al. (2004). Depressive symptoms in elderly patients predict poor adjustment after somatic events. *American Journal of Geriatric Psychiatry, 12,* 57-64.

Dennis, M.S., & Lindesay, J. (1995). Suicide in the elderly–The United Kingdom Perspective. *International Psychogeriatrics, 7,* 263-274.

Devanand, D.P., Kim, M.K., Paykina, N., & Sackeim, H.A. (2002). Adverse life events in elderly patients with major depression or dysthymic disorder and in healthy-control subjects. *American Journal of Geriatric Psychiatry, 10*(3), 265-74.

Dietrich, A.J., Oxman, T.E., Williams, J.W. Jr., Kroenke, K., Schulberg, H.C., Bruce, M., & Barry, S.L. (2004). Going to scale: Re-engineering systems for primary care treatment of depression. *Annals of Family Medicine, 2*(4), 301-4.

Doraiswamy, P.M., Khan, Z.M., Donahue, R.M.J., & Richard, N.E. (2002). The spectrum of quality-of-life impairments in recurrent geriatric depression. *Journal of Gerontology: Medical Sciences, 57,* M134-M137.

Doraiswamy, P.M., Krishnan, K.R., Oxman, T., Jenkyn, L.R., Coffey, D.J., Burt, T., & Clary, C.M. (2003). Does antidepressant therapy improve cognition in elderly depressed patients? *Journals of Gerontology Series A-Biological Sciences & Medical Sciences, 58*(12), M1137-44.

Dunner, D.L. (2003). Treatment considerations for depression in the elderly. *CNS Spectrums, 8, Suppl 3,* 14-9.

Dwight-Johnson, M. et al. (2000). Treatment preferences among depressed primary care patients. *JGIM, 15,* 527-534.

Dwight-Johnson, M. et al. (2001). Can quality improvement programs for depression in primary care address patient preferences for treatment? *Medical Care, 39*(9), 934-944.

Dwight-Johnson, M., Lagomasino, I.T., Aisenberg, E., & Hay, J. (2004). Using conjoint analysis to assess depression treatment preferences among low-income Latinos. *Psychiatric Services, 55,* 934-936.

Dwight-Johnson, M., Ell, K., & Jiuan-Lee, P. (2005). Can collaborative care address the needs of low-income Latinas with comorbid depression and cancer? Results from a randomized pilot study. *Psychosomatics,* 46(3) 224-32.

Eggar, R., Spencer, A., Anderson, D., & Hiller, L. (2002). Views of elderly patients on cardiopulmonary resuscitation before and after treatment for depression. *International Journal of Geriatric Psychiatry, 17*(2), 170-4.

Ell, K., & Enguidanos, S. (2004). Evidence-based Depression Care for Elders in Home Health & Geriatric Care Management. National Gerontological Social Work Conference, Anaheim, CA, March.

Ell, K., Unützer, J., Aranda, M., Sanchez, K., & Lee, P.J. (2004). Routine PHQ-9 Depression Screening in Home Health Care: Depression Prevalence, Clinical and Treatment Characteristics. Unpublished Paper.

Engberg, S., Sereika, S., Weber, E., Engberg, R., McDowell, B.J., & Reynolds, C.F. (2001). Prevalence and recognition of depressive symptoms among homebound older adults with urinary incontinence. *Journal of Geriatric Psychiatry & Neurology, 14,* 130-139.

Evans, D.L., Staab, J.P., Petitto, J.M., Morrison, M.F., Szuba, M.P., Ward, H.E. et al. (1999) Depression in the medical setting: Biopsychological interactions and treatment considerations. *Journal of Clinical Psychiatry, 60 Suppl 4,* 40-55.

Fazzi, R.A., & Wright, K. (2003). Improving OASIS accuracy: A national effort. *Caring Magazine, 23,* 52-56.

Fischer, L.R., Wei, F., Solberg, L.I., Rush, W.A., & Heinrich, R.L. (2003). Treatment of elderly and other adult patients for depression in primary care. *Journal of the American Geriatrics Society, 51*(11), 1554-62.

Flaherty, J.H., McBride, M., Marzouk, S., Miller, D.K., Chien, N., Hanchett, M. et al. (1998). Decreasing hospitalization rates for older home care patients with symptoms of depression. *Journal of the American Geriatrics Society, 46,* 31-38.

Flint, A.J. (2002). The complexity and challenge of non-major depression in late life. *American Journal of Geriatric Psychiatry, 10,* 229-232.

Frank, R.G., Huskamp, H.A., & Pincus, H.A. (2003). Aligning incentives in the treatment of depression in primary care with evidence-based practice. *Psychiatric Services, 54,* 682-687.

Gallo, J.J., Cooper-Patrick, L., & Lesikar, S. (1998). Depressive symptoms of whites and African Americans aged 60 years and older. *Journal of Gerentology: Psychological Sciences & Social Science, 53,* 277-286.

Gallo, J.J., Zubritsky, C., Maxwell, J., Nazar, M., Bogner, H.R., Quijano, L.M. et al. & PRISM-E Investigators. (2004). Primary care clinicians evaluate integrated and referral models of behavioral health care for older adults: Results from a multisite effectiveness trial (PRISM-e). *Annals of Family Medicine, 2,* 305-9.

Ganguli, G. (2003). Consumers Devise Drug Cost-Cutting Measures: Medical and Legal Issues to Consider. *Health Care Manager, 22,* 275-281.

Geerlings, S.W., Beekman, A.T., Deeg, D.J., Twisk, J.W., & Van Tilburg, W. (2002). Duration and severity of depression predict mortality in older adults in the community. *Psychological Medicine, 32,* 609-618.

Gerrity, M.S., Williams, J.W., Dietrich, A.J., & Olson, A.L. (2001). Identifying physicians likely to benefit from depression education: A challenge for health care organizations. *Medical Care, 39*(8), 856-66.

Goldman, B., Balgobin, S., Bish, R., Lee, R.H., McCue, S., Morrison, M.H. et al. (2004). Nurse educators are key to a best practices implementation program. *Geriatric Nursing, 25,* 171-174.

Goldman, D. P., Joyce, G. F., Escarce, J.J., Pace, J. E., Solomon, M. D., Laouri, M. et al. (2004). Pharmacy Benefits and the Use of Drugs by the Chronically Ill. *Journal of the American Medical Association, 291,* 2344-2350.

González, H.M., Haan, M.N., & Hinton, L. (2001). Acculturation and the prevalence of depression in older Mexican Americans: Baseline results of the Sacramento area Latino study on aging. *Journal of the American Geriatrics Society, 49,* 948-953.

Goulding, M.R. (2004). Inappropriate medication prescribing for elderly ambulatory care patients. *Archives of Internal Medicine, 164,* 305-12.

Green-Hennessy, S., & Hennessy, K.D. (1999). Demographic differences in medication use among individuals with self-reported major depression. *Psychiatric Services, 50,* 257-9.

Groh, C.J., & Hoes, M.L. (2003). Practice methods among nurse practitioners treating depressed women. *Journal of the American Academy of Nurse Practitioners, 15,* 130-136.

Gum, A., & Areán, P.A. (2004). Current status of psychotherapy for mental disorders in the elderly. *Current Psychological Reports, 6,* 32-38.

Harman, J.S., Crystal, S., Walkup, J., & Olfson, M. (2003). Trends in elderly patients' office visits for the treatment of depression according to physician specialty: 1985-1999. *Journal of Behavioral Health Services & Research, 30*(3), 332-41.

Harman, J.S., Edlund, M.J., & Fortney, J.C. (2004). Disparities in the adequacy of depression treatment in the United States. *Psychiatric Services, 55,* 1379-1385.

Harpole, L.H., Stechuchak, K.M., Saur, C.D., Steffens, D.C., Unützer, J., & Oddone, E. (2003). Implementing a disease management intervention for depression in primary care: A random work sampling study. *General Hospital Psychiatry, 25*(4), 238-45.

Haverkamp, R., Areán, P., Hegel, M.T., & Unützer, J. (2004). Problem-solving treatment for complicated depression in late life: A case study in primary care. *Perspectives in Psychiatric Care, 40,* 45-52.

Hayes, D. (2004). Recent developments in antidepressant therapy in special populations. *American Journal of Managed Care, 10(6 Suppl),* S179-85.

Hays, J.C., Steffens, D.C., Flint, E.P., Bosworth, H.B., & George, L.K. (2001). Does social support buffer functional decline in elderly patients with unipolar depression? *American Journal of Psychiatry, 158,* 1850-1855.

Hendrie, H.C., Callahan, C.M., Levitt, E.E., Hui, S.L., Musick, B., Austrom, M.G. et al. (1995). Prevalence rates of major depressive disorders: The effects of varying the diagnostic criteria in an older primary care population. *American Journal of Geriatric Psychology, 5,* 119-131.

Henriksson, M.M., Marttunen, M.J., Isometsä, E.T., Heikkinen, M.E., Aro, H.M., Kuoppasalmi, K.I., & Lönnqvist, J.K. (1995). Mental disorders in elderly suicide. *International Psychogeriatrics, 7,* 275-286.

Holman, H., & Lorig, K. (2004). Patient self-management: A key to effectiveness and efficiency in care of chronic disease. *Public Health Reports, 119*(3), 239-43.

Huffman, G.B. (2002). Evaluating and treating unintentional weight loss in the elderly. *American Family Physician, 65,* 640-650.

Hunkeler, E.M., Meresman, J.F., Hargreaves, W.A., Fireman, B., Berman, W.H., Kirsch, A.J. et al. (2000). Efficacy of nurse telehealth care and peer support in augmenting treatment of depression in primary care. *Archives of Family Medicine, 9*(8), 700-8.

Improving Chronic Illness Care ICIC (2002a): The Chronic Care Model: Model Components: Overview of the Chronic Care Model. www.improvingchroniccare.org/change/model/components.html

Johnson, R.L., Saha, S., Arbelaez, J.J., Beach, M.C., & Cooper, L.A. (2004). Racial and ethnic differences in patient perceptions of bias and cultural competence in health care. *Journal of General Internal Medicine, 19,* 101-110.

Jongenelis, K., Pot, A.M., Eises, A.M.H., Beekman, A.T.F., Kluiter, H., & Ribbe, M.W. (2004). Prevalence and risk indicators of depression in elderly nursing home patients: The AGED study. *Journal of Affective Disorders, 83,* 135-142.

Jorm, A.F. (1998). Epidemiology of mental disorders in old age. *Current Opinion Psychiatry, 11,* 405-409.

Juurlink, D.N., Herrmann, N., Szalai, J.P., Kopp, A., & Redelmeier, D.A. (2004). Medical illness and the risk of suicide in the elderly. *Archives of Internal Medicine, 164,* 1179-1184.

Katon, W.J., Lin, E., Russo, J., & Unützer, J. (2003). Increased medical costs of a population-based sample of depressed elderly patients. *Archives of General Psychiatry, 60,* 897-903.

Katz, I.R. (1996). On the inseparability of mental and physical health in aged persons: Lessons from depression and medical comorbidity. *American Journal of Geriatric Psychiatry, 4,* 1-16.

Kindy, D. (2003). Ongoing primary care intervention increased remission and emotional and physical role functioning in major depression. *Evidence-Based Nursing, 6,* 86.

Knauper, B., & Wittchen, H.U. (1994). Diagnosing major depression in the elderly: Evidence for response bias in standardized diagnostic interviews? *Journal of Psychiatric Research, 8,* 147-164.

Koenig, H.G., & George, L.K. (1998). Depression and physical disability outcomes in depressed medically ill hospitalized older adults. *American Journal of Geriatric Psychiatry, 6,* 230-247.

Koenig, H.G., & Kutchibhatla, M. (1999). Use of health services by medically ill depressed elderly patients after hospital discharge. *American Journal of Geriatric Psychiatry, 7,* 48-56.

Koenig, H.G., Gittelman, D., Branski, S., Brown, S., Stone, P., & Ostrow, B. (1998). Depressive symptoms in elderly medical-surgical patients hospitalized in community settings. *American Journal of Geriatric Psychiatry, 6*(1), 14-23.

Kohn, R., Goldsmith, E., & Sedgwick, T.W. (2002). Treatment of homebound mentally ill elderly patients: The multidisciplinary psychiatric mobile team. *American Journal of Geriatric Psychiatry, 10,* 469-475.

Koike, A.K., Unützer, J., & Wells, K.B. (2002). Improving the care for depression in patients with comorbid medical illness. *American Journal of Psychiatry, 159,* 1738-1745.

Kraaij, V., Arensman, E., & Spinhoven, P. (2002). Negative life events and depression in elderly persons: A meta-analysis. *Journals of Gerontology Series B-Psychological Sciences & Social Sciences, 57*(1), 87-94.

Kroenke, K., & Spitzer, R.L. (2002). The PHQ-9: A new depression diagnostic and severity measure. *Psychiatric Annual, 32,* 509-515.

Kroenke, K., Spitzer, R.L., & Williams, J.B. (2001). The PHQ-9: Validity of a brief depression severity measure. *Journal of General Internal Medicine, 169,* 606-13.

Kunik, M.E., Braun, U., Stanley, M.A., Wristers, K., Molinari, V., Stoebner, D., & Orengo, C.A. (2001). One session cognitive behavioural therapy for elderly patients with chronic obstructive pulmonary disease. *Psychological Medicine, 31*(4), 717-23.

Kurlowicz, L.H. (2003). Depression in older adults. In: Mezey M., Fulmer T., Abraham I., Zwicker D.A., editor(s). *Geriatric nursing protocols for best practice. 2nd ed.* New York (NY): Springer Publishing Company, Inc. pp. 185-206.

Langa, K.M., Valenstein, M.A., Fendrick, A.M., Kabeto, M.U., & Vijan, S. (2004). Extent and cost of informal caregiving for older Americans with symptoms of depression. *American Journal of Psychiatry, 161,* 857-63.

Larson, J.S., Chernoff, R., & Sweet-Holp, T.J. (2004). An evaluation of provider educational needs in geriatric care. *Evaluation & the Health Professions, 27,* 95-103.

Lavretsky, H., & Kuman, A. (2002). Clinically significant non-major depression: Old concepts, new insights. *American Journal of Geriatric Psychiatry, 10,* 239-255.

Lavretsky, H., Bastani, R., Gould, R., Huang, D., Llorente, M., Maxwell, A., & Jarvik, L. (2002). UPBEAT Collaborative Group. Unified Psychogeriatric Biopsychological Evaluation and Treatment. Predictors of two-year mortality in a prospective "UPBEAT" study of elderly veterans with comorbid medical and psychiatric symptoms. *American Journal of Geriatric Psychiatry, 10,* 458-68.

Lebowitz, B.D., Pearson, J.L., Schneider, L.S., Reynolds, C.F., Alexopoulow, G.S., Bruce, M.L. et al. (1997). Diagnosis and treatment of depression in late life: Consensus statement update. *JAMA, 278,* 1186-1190.

Lenze, E.J. (2003). Comorbidity of depression and anxiety in the elderly. *Current Psychiatry Reports, 5,* 62-67.

Lenze, E.J., Mulsant, B.H., Dew, M.A., Shear, M.K., Houck, P., Pollock, B.G., & Reynolds, C.F. 3rd. (2003). Good treatment outcomes in late-life depression with comorbid anxiety. *Journal of Affective Disorders, 77,* 247-54.

Lin, E. H., Katon, W.J., Simon, G.E., VonKorff, M., Bush, T.M., Rutter, C.M. et al. (1997). Achieving guidelines for the treatment of depression in primary care: Is physician education enough? *Medical Care, 35,* 831-842.

Lin, E.H., Katon, W., Von Korff, M., Tan, L., Williams, J.W. Jr., Kroenke, K. et al. (2003). IMPACT Investigators: Effect of improving depression care on pain and functional outcomes among older adults with arthritis: A randomized controlled trial. *JAMA, 290*, 2428-9.

Lin, E.H., Von Korff, M., Ludman, E.J., Rutter, C., Bush, T.M., Simon, G.E. et al. (2003). Enhancing adherence to prevent depression relapse in primary care. *General Hospital Psychiatry, 25*, 303-10.

Lish, J.D., Zimmerman, M., Farber, N.J., Lush, D.T., Kuzma, M.A., & Plescia, G. (1996). Suicide screening in a primary care setting at a Veterans Affairs Medical Center. *Psychosomatics, 37*, 413-424.

Löwe, B., Gräfe, K., Zipfel, S., Witte, S., Loerch, B., & Herzog, W. (2004). Diagnosing ICD-10 depressive episodes: Superior criterion validity of the Patient Health Questionnaire. *Psychotherapy & Psychosomatics, 73*(6), 386-90.

Löwe, B., Kroenke, K., Herzog, W., & Gräfe, K. (2004). Measuring depression outcome with a brief self-report instrument: Sensitivity to change of the Patient Health Questionnaire (PHQ-9). *Journal of Affective Disorders, 81*, 61-66.

Löwe, B., Spitzer, R.L., Gräfe, K., Kroenke, K., Quenter, A., Zipfel, S. et al. (2004). Comparative validity of three screening questionnaires for DSM-IV depressive disorders and physicians' diagnoses. *Journal of Affective Disorders, 78*, 131-140.

Löwe, B., Unützer, J., Callahan, C.M., Perkins, A.J., & Kroenke, K. (2004). Monitoring depression treatment outcomes with the PHQ-9. *Medical Care, 42*(12), 1194-201.

Luber, M.P., Meyers, B.S., Williams-Russo, P.G., Hollenberg, J.P., DiDomenico, T.N., Charlson, M.E., & Alexopoulos, G.S. (2001). Depression and service utilization in elderly primary care patients. *American Journal of Geriatric Psychiatry, 9*, 169-176.

Lyness, J.M. (2004). Treatment of depressive conditions in later life. *JAMA, 291*, 1626-1627.

Lyness, J.M., Caine, E.D., King, D.A., Conwell, Y., Duberstein, P.R., & Cox, C. (2002). Depressive disorders and symptoms in older primary care patients: One-year outcomes. *American Journal of Geriatric Psychiatry, 10*, 275-282.

Lyness, J.M., Cox, C., Curry, J., Conwell, Y., King, D.A., & Caine, E.D. (1995). Older age and the underreporting of depressive symptoms. *Journal of American Geriatrics Society, 43*, 216-221.

Maidment, R., Livingston, G., & Katona, C. (2002). 'Just keep taking the tablets': Adherence to antidepressant treatment in older people in primary care. *International Journal of Geriatric Psychiatry, 17*, 752-757.

Marwaha, S., & Livingston, G. (2002). Stigma, racism or choice. Why do depressed ethnic elders avoid psychiatrists? *Journal of Affective Disorders, 72*, 257-265.

Mayall, E., Oathamshaw, S., Lovell, K., & Pusey, H. (2004). Development and piloting of a multidisciplinary training course for detecting and managing depression in the older person. *Journal of Psychiatry and Mental Health Nursing, 11*, 165-171.

McAvay, G.J., Bruce, M.L., Raue, P.J., & Brown, E. (2004). Depression in elderly homecare patients: Patient versus informant reports. *Psychological Medicine, 34*(8), 1507-17

McDonald, M.V., Passik, S.D., Dugan, W., Rosenfeld, B., Theobald, D.E., & Edgerton, S. (1999). Nurses' recognition of depression in their patients with cancer. *Oncology Nursing Forum, 26*, 593-599.

Mehta, K.M., Yaffe, K., Langa, K.M., Sands, L., Whooley, M.A., & Covinsky, K.E. (2003). Additive effects of cognitive function and depressive symptoms on mortality in elderly community-living adults. *Journal of Gerontology Series A-Biological Sciences & Medical Sciences, 58*, M461-7.

Melfi, C.A., Croghan, T.W., & Hanna, M.P. (1999). Access to treatment for depression in a Medicaid population. *Journal of Health Care for the Poor & Underserved, 10*, 201-15.

Melfi, C.A., Croghan, T.W., Hanna, M.P., & Robinson, R.L. (2000). Racial variation in antidepressant treatment in a Medicaid population. *Journal of Clinical Psychiatry, 61*, 16-21.

Meresman, J.F., Hunkeler, E.M., Hargreaves, W.A., Kirsch, A.J., Robinson, P., Green, A. et al. (2003). A case report: Implementing a nurse telecare program for treating depression in primary care. *Psychiatric Quarterly, 74*, 61-73.

Miller, M.D., Cornes, C., Frank, E., Ehrenpreis, L., Silberman, R., Schlernitzauer, M.A. et al. (2001). Interpersonal psychotherapy for late-life depression: Past, present, and future. *Journal of Psychotherapy Practice & Research, 10*(4), 231-8.

Miller, M.D., Frank, E., Cornes, C., Houck, P.R., & Reynolds, C.F. 3rd. (2003). The value of maintenance interpersonal psychotherapy (IPT) in older adults with different IPT foci. *American Journal of Geriatric Psychiatry, 11*(1), 97-102.

Mills, T.L., Alea, N.L., & Cheong, J.A. (2004). Differences in the indicators of depressive symptoms among a community sample of African-American and Caucasian older adults. *Community Mental Health Journal, 40*, 309-331.

Miranda, J., Duan, N., Sherbourne, C., Schoenbaum, M., Lagomasino, I., Jackson-Triche, M., & Wells, K.B. (2003). Improving care for minorities: Can quality improvement interventions improve care and outcomes for depressed minorities? Results of a randomized, controlled trial. *Health Services Research, 38*, 613-30.

Mojtabai, R., & Olfson, M. (2004). Major depression in community-dwelling middle-aged and older adults: Prevalence and 2- and 4-year follow-up symptoms. *Psychological Medicine, 34*, 623-634.

Moser, D.K. (2002). Psychosocial factors and their association with clinical outcomes in patients with heart failure: Why clinicians do not seem to care. *European Journal of Cardiovascular Nursing, 1*(3), 183-8.

Mueller, T.I., Kohn, R. Leventhal, N., Leon, A.C., Solomon, D., Coryell, W. et al. (2004). The course of depression in elderly patients. *American Journal of Geriatric Psychiatry, 12*(1), 22-9.

Mulsant, B.H., Whyte, E., Lenze, E.J., Lotrich, F., Karp, J.F., Pollock, B.G., & Reynolds, C.F. 3rd. (2003). Achieving long-term optimal outcomes in geriatric depression and anxiety. *CNS Spectrums, 8(12 Suppl 3)*, 27-34.

Nolan, P., Murray, E., & Dallender, J. (1999). Practice nurses' perceptions of services for clients with psychological problems in primary care. *International Journal of Nursing Studies, 36*, 97-104.

Oishi, S.M., Shoai, R., Katon, W., Callahan, C., Unützer, J., Arean, P. et al. (2003). Improving Mood: Promoting Access to Collaborative Treatment Investigators. Impacting late life depression: Integrating a depression intervention into primary care. *Psychiatric Quarterly, 74*(1), 75-89.

Oxman, T.E. et al. (2002). A three-component model for reengineering systems for the treatment of depression in primary care. *Psychosomatics, 43*, 441-450.

Oxman, T.E.,Dietrich, A.J., & Schulberg, H.C. (2003). The depression care manager and mental health specialist as collaborators within primary care. *American Journal of Geriatric Psychiatry, 11*(5), 507-16.

Pearson, B., Katz, S.E., Soucie, V., Hunkeler, E., Meresman, J., Rooney, T., & Amick, B.C. 3rd. (2003). Evidence-based care for depression in Maine: Dissemination of the Kaiser Permanente Nurse Telecare Program. *Psychiatric Quarterly, 74*(1), 91-102.

Penninx, B. W., Guralnik, J.M., Ferrucci, L., Simonsick, E.M., Deeg, D., & Wallace, R.B. (1998). Depressive symptoms and physical decline in community-dwelling older persons. *JAMA, 279*, 1720-1726.

Peterson, L.E. (2004). Strengthening condition-specific evidence-based home health care practice. *Journal for Healthcare Quality, 26*, 10-18.

Pfaff, J.J., & Almeida, O.P. (2004). Identifying suicidal ideation among older adults in a general practice setting. *Journal of Affective Disorders, 83*, 73-7.

Pignone, M.P., Gaynes, B.N., Rushton, J.L., Burchell, C.M., Orleans, C.T., Mulrow, C.D. et al. (2002). Screening for depression in adults: A summary of the evidence for the U.S. Preventive Services Task Force. *Annals of Internal Medicine, 136*, 765-776.

Pirraglia, P.A., Rosen, A.B., Hermann, R.C., Olchanski, N.V., & Neumann, P. (2004). Cost-utility analysis studies of depression management: A systematic review. *American Journal of Psychiatry, 161*, 2155-2162.

Posternak, M.A., & Zimmerman, M. (2003). How accurate are patients in reporting their antidepressant treatment history? *Journal of Affective Disorders, 75*, 115-124.

Prabhakaran, P., & Butler, R. (2002). What are older peoples' experiences of taking antidepressants? *Journal of Affective Disorders, 70*, 319-322.

Preville, M., Cote, G., Boyer, R., & Hebert, R. (2004). Detection of depression and anxiety disorders by home care nurses. *Aging & Mental Health, 8*, 400-9.

Proudfoot, J., Goldberg, D., Mann, A., Everitt, B., Marks, I., & Gray, J.A. (2003). Computerized, interactive, multimedia cognitive-behavioural program for anxiety and depression in general practice. *Psychological Medicine, 33*(2), 217-27.

Pulska, T., Pahkala, K., Laippala, P., & Kivela, S.L. (1998). Survival of elderly Finns suffering from dysthymic disorder: A community study. *Social Psychiatry & Psychiatric Epidemiology, 33*, 319-325.

Ranga, K., Krishnan, R., Delong, M., Kraemer, H., Carney, R., Spiegel, D. et al. (2002). Comorbidity of depression with other medical diseases in the elderly. *Biological Psychiatry, 52*, 559-588.

Ranga, R.K., George, L.K., Peiper, C.F., Jiang, W., Arias, R., Look, A., & O'Connor, C. (1998). Depression and social support in elderly patients with cardiac disease. *American Heart Journal, 136*, 491-495.

Rao, A., & Cohen, J.J. (2004). Symptom management in the elderly cancer patient: Fatigue, pain, and depression. *Journal of National Cancer Institute Monographs, 32*, 150-157.

Raue, P.J., Brown, E.L., & Bruce, M.L. (2002). Assessing behavioral health using OASIS: Part 1 Depression and suicidality. *Home Healthcare Nurse, 20*, 154-161.

Raue, P.J., Meyers, B.S., McAvay, G.J., Brown, E.L., Keohane, D.J., & Bruce, M.E. (2003). One-month stability of depression among elderly home-care patients. *American Journal of Geriatric Psychiatry, 11(5), 543-50.*

Reuben, D.B. (2002). Organizational interventions to improve health outcomes of older persons. *Medical Care, 40,* 416-428.

Reynolds, C.F. 3rd, Frank, E., Perel, J.M., Imber, S.D., Cornes, C., Miller, M.D. et al. (1999). Nortriptyline and interpersonal psychotherapy as maintenance therapies for recurrent major depression: A randomized controlled trial in patients older than 59 years. *JAMA, 281,* 39-45.

Reynolds, C.F. 3rd, Miller, M.D., Pasternak, R.E., Frank, E., Perel, J.M., Cornes, C. et al. (1999). Treatment of bereavement-related major depressive episodes in later life: A controlled study of acute and continuation treatment with nortriptyline and interpersonal psychotherapy. *American Journal of Psychiatry, 156,* 202-208.

Reynolds, C.F., Dew, M.A., Frank, E., Begley, A.E., Miller, M.D., Cornes, C. et al. (1998). Effects of age at onset of first lifetime episode of recurrent major depression on treatment response and illness course in elderly patients. *American Journal of Psychiatry, 155,* 795-799.

Reynolds, C.F., Frank, E., Perel, J. et al. (1995). Maintenance therapies for late life recurrent major depression: Research and review circa 1995. *International Psychogeriatrics, 7 (suppl),* 27-40.

Rihmer, Z. (1996). Strategies of suicide prevention: Focus on health care. *Journal of Affective Disorders, 39,* 83-91.

Rihmer, Z., Rutz, W., & Pihlgren, H. (1995). Depression and suicide on Gotland: An intensive study of all suicides before and after a depression-training program for general practitioners. *Journal of Affective Disorders, 35,* 147-152.

Roeloffs, C., Sherbourne, C., Unützer, J., Fink, A., Tang, L., & Wells, K.B. (2003). Stigma and depression among primary care patients. *General Hospital Psychiatry, 25(5),* 311-5.

Rosen, J., Mulsant, B.H., Kollar, M., Kastango, K.B., Mazumdar, S., & Fox, D. (2002). Mental health training for nursing home staff using computer-based interactive video: A 6-month randomized trial. *Journal of the American Medical Directors Association, 3,* 291-296.

Rost, K., Nutting, P., Smith, J., Werner, J., & Duan, N. (2001). Improving depression outcomes in community primary care practice: A randomized trial of the QuEST intervention. *JGIM, 16,* 143-149.

Rutz, W., von Knorring, L., & Wålinder, J. (1989). Frequency of suicide on Gotland after systematic postgraduate education of general practitioners. *Acta Psychiatrica Scandinavica, 80,* 151-154.

Sable, J.A., Dunn, L.B., & Zisook, S. (2002). Late-life depression: How to identify its symptoms and provide effective treatment. *Geriatrics, 57,* 18-35.

Salzman, C. (1995). Medication adherence in the elderly. *Journal of Clinical Psychiatry, 56,* 18-22.

Salzman, C., Wong, E., & Wright, B.C. (2002). Drug and ECT treatment of depression in the elderly, 1996-2001: A literature review. *Biological Psychiatry, 52,* 265-284.

Sambamoorthi, U., Olfson, M., Walkup, J.T., & Crystal, S. (2003). Diffusion of new generation antidepressant treatment among elderly diagnosed with depression. *Medical Care, 41(1),* 180-94.

Sanderson, K., Andrews, G., Corry, J., & Lapsley, H. (2003). Reducing the burden of affective disorders: Is evidence-based health care affordable?. *Journal of Affective Disorders, 77*(2), 109-25.

Schoenbaum, M., Miranda, J., Sherbourne, C., Duan, N., & Wells, K. (2004). Cost-effectiveness of interventions for depressed Latinos. *Journal of Mental Health Policy & Economics, 7*, 69-76.

Schoenbaum, M., Unützer, J., Sherbourne, C., Duan, N., Rubenstein, L. V., Miranda, J. et al. (2001). Cost-effectiveness of practice-initiated quality improvement for depression: Results of a randomized controlled trial. *JAMA, 286*(11), 1325-30.

Schulberg, H.C., Bruce, M.L., Lee, P.W., Williams, J.W. Jr., & Dietrich, A.J. (2004). Preventing suicide in primary care patients: The primary care physician's role. *General Hospital Psychiatry, 26*(5), 337-45.

Schulz, R., Drayer, R.A., & Rollman, B.L. (2002). Depression as a risk factor for non-suicide mortality in the elderly. *Biological Psychiatry, 52*, 205-225.

Sclar, D.A., Robison, L.M., Skaer, T.L., & Galin, R.S. (1999). Ethnicity and the prescribing of antidepressant pharmacotherapy: 1992-1995. *Harvard Review of Psychiatry, 7*(1), 29-36.

Scocco, P., & Frank, E. (2002). Interpersonal psychotherapy as augmentation treatment in depressed elderly responding poorly to antidepressant drugs: A case series. *Psychotherapy & Psychosomatics, 71*(6), 357-61.

Serby, M., & Yu, M. (2003). Overview: Depression in the elderly. *Mount Sinai Journal of Medicine, 70*, 38-44.

Sewitch, M.J., McCusker, J., Dendukuri, N., & Yaffe, M.J. (2004). Depression in frail elders: Impact on family caregivers. *International Journal of Geriatric Psychiatry, 19*, 655-65.

Sheeran, T., Brown, E.L., Nassisi, P., & Bruce, M.L. (2004). Does depression predict falls among home health patients? Using a clinical-research partnership to improve the quality of geriatric care. *Home Healthcare Nurse, 22*, 384-389.

Sheikh, J.I., Cassidy, E.L., Doraiswamy, P.M., Salomon, R.M., Hornig, M., Holland, P.J. et al. (2004). Efficacy, safety, and tolerability of sertraline in patients with late-life depression and comorbid medical illness. *Journal of American Geriatrics Society, 52*, 86-92.

Sherbourne, C.D., Wells, K.B., Duan, N., Miranda, J., Unützer, J., Jaycox, L. et al. (2001). Long-term effectiveness of disseminating quality improvement for depression in primary care. *Archives of General Psychiatry, 58*(7), 696-703.

Simon, G.E., Katon, W.J., VonKorff, M., Unützer, J., Lin, E.H.B., Walker, E.A. et al. (2001). Cost-effectiveness of a collaborative care program for primary care patients with persistent depression. *American Journal of Psychiatry, 158*, 1638-1644.

Simon, G.E., Ludman, E.J., Tutty, S., Operskalski, B., & Von Korff, M. (2004). Telephone psychotherapy and telephone care management for primary care patients starting antidepressant treatment: A randomized controlled trial. *JAMA, 292*, 935-42.

Simon, G.E., Von Korff, M., Ludman, E.J., Katon, W.J., Rutter, C., Unützer, J. et al. (2002). Cost-effectiveness of a program to prevent depression relapse in primary care. *Medical Care, 40*(10), 941-50.

Sirey, J.A., Bruce, M.L., Alexopoulos, G.S., Perlick, D.A., Friedman, S.J., & Meyers B.S. (2001). Stigma as a barrier to recovery: Perceived stigma and patient-rated severity of illness as predictors of antidepressant drug adherence. *Psychiatric Services, 52*(12), 1615-20.

Sirey, J.A., Bruce, M.L., Alexopoulos, G.S., Perlick, D.A., Raue, P., Friedman, S.J., & Meyers, B.S. (2001). Perceived stigma as a predictor of treatment discontinuation in young and older outpatients with depression. *American Journal of Psychiatry, 158*(3), 479-81.

Skaer, T.L., Sclar, D.A., Robison, L.M., & Galin, R.S. (2000). Trends in the rate of depressive illness and use of antidepressant pharmacotherapy by ethnicity/race: An assessment of office-based visits in the United States, 1992-1997. *Clinical Therapeutics, 22*(12), 1575-89.

Smith, L., Walker, A., & Gilhooly, K. (2004). Clinical guidelines of depression: A qualitative study of GPs' views. *Journal of Family Practice, 53*(7), 556-61.

Sommer, B.R., Fenn, H., Pompei, P., DeBattista, C., Lembke, A., Wang, P., & Flores, B. (2003) Safety of antidepressants in the elderly. *Expert Opinion on Drug Safety, 2*(4), 367-83.

Sonnenberg, C.M., Beekman, A.T., Deeg, D.J., & Tilburg, V. (2003). Drug treatment in depressed elderly in the Dutch community. *International Journal of Geriatric Psychiatry, 18*(2), 99-104.

Soumerai, S.B. (1998). Principles and uses of academic detailing to improve the management of psychiatric disorders. *International Journal of Psychiatry in Medicine, 28*, 81-86.

Spitzer, R.L., Kroenke, K., & Williams, J.B. (1999). Validation and utility of a self-report version of PRIME-MD: The PHQ primary care study. Primary Care Evaluation of Mental Disorders. Patient Health Questionnaire. *JAMA, 282*, 1737-44.

Steffens, D.C., Skoog, I., Norton, M.C., Hart, A.D. Tschanz, J.T., Plassman et al. (2000). Prevalence of depression and its treatment in an elderly population: The Cache County study. *Archives of General Psychiatry, 57*, 601-607.

Stein, M.B., & Barrett-Connor, E. (2002). Quality of life in older adults receiving medications for anxiety, depression, or insomnia: Findings from a community-based study. *American Journal of Geriatric Psychiatry, 10*(5), 568-74.

Streim, J.E., Oslin, D.W., Katz, I.R., Smith, B.D., DiFilippo, S., Cooper, T.B., & Ten Have, T. (2000). Drug treatment of depression in frail elderly nursing home residents. *American Journal of Geriatric Psychiatry, 8*(2), 150-9.

Suominen, K., Henriksson, M., Isometsa, E., Conwell, Y., Heila, H., & Lonnqvist, J. (2003). Nursing home suicides–a psychological autopsy study. *International Journal of Geriatric Psychiatry, 18*, 1095-101.

Suominen, K., Isometsa, E., & Lonnqvist, J. (2004). Elderly suicide attempters with depression are often diagnosed only after the attempt. *International Journal of Geriatric Psychiatry, 19*, 35-40.

Symons, L., Tylee, A., Mann, A., Jones, R., Plummer, S., Walker, M. et al. (2004). Improving access to depression care: Descriptive report of a multidisciplinary primary care pilot service. *British Journal of General Practice, 54*(506), 679-83.

Szanto, K., Mulsant, B.H., Houck, P., Dew, M.A., & Reynolds, C.F. 3rd. (2003). Occurrence and course of suicidality during short-term treatment of late-life depression. *Archives of General Psychiatry, 60*, 610-617.

Taylor, M.P., Reynolds, C.F., 3rd, Frank, E., Cornes, C., Miller, M.D., & Stack, J.A. (1999). Which elderly patients remain well on maintenance interpersonal psychotherapy alone? Report from Pittsburgh study of maintenance therapies in late life depression. *Depression & Anxiety, 10*, 55-60.

Taylor, W.D., & Doraiswamy, P.M. (2004). A systematic review of antidepressant placebo-controlled trials for geriatric depression: Limitations of current data and directions for the future. *Neuropsychopharmacology, 29*, 2285-99.

Thomas, L., Mulsant, B.H., Solano, F.X., Black, A.M., Bensasi, S., Flynn, T. et al. (2002). Response speed and rate of remission in primary and specialty care of elderly patients with depression. *American Journal of Geriatric Psychiatry, 10*, 583-9.

Thomas, P., Hazif-Thomas, C., & Clement, J.P. (2003). Influence of antidepressant therapies on weight and appetite in the elderly. *Journal of Nutrition, Health & Aging, 7*(3), 166-70.

Thompson, L.W., Coon, D.W., Gallagher-Thompson, D., Sommer, B.R., & Koin, D. (2001). Comparison of desipramine and cognitive/behavioral therapy in the treatment of elderly outpatients with mild-to-moderate depression. *American Journal of Geriatric Psychiatry, 9*(3), 225-40.

Torrisi, D., & McDaniel, H. (2003). Better outcomes for depressed patients. *The Nurse Practitioner, 28*, 32-38.

Uncapher, H., & Areán, P.A. (2000). Physicians are less willing to treat suicidal ideation in older patients. *Journal of the American Geriatrics Society, 48*(2), 188-92.

Unützer, J. (2002). Diagnosis and treatment of older adults with depression in primary care. *Biological Psychiatry, 52*, 285-292.

Unützer, J., Ferrell, B., Lin, E.H., & Marmon, T. (2004). Pharmacotherapy of pain in depressed older adults. *Journal of American Geriatrics Society, 52*, 1916-22.

Unützer, J., Katon, W., Callahan, C.M., Williams Jr., J.W., Hunkeler, E., Harpole, L. et al. (2002). Collaborative care management of late-life depression in the primary care setting: A randomized controlled trial. *JAMA, 288*, 2836-2845.

Unützer, J., Katon, W., Callahan, C.M., Williams, J.W. Jr., Hunkeler, E., Harpole, L. et al. (2003). Depression treatment in a sample of 1,801 depressed older adults in primary care. *Journal of the American Geriatrics Society, 51*(4), 505-14.

Unützer, J., Katon, W., Sullivan, M., & Miranda, J. (1999). Treating depressed older adults in primary care: Narrowing the gap between efficacy and effectiveness. *The Millbank Quarterly, 77*, 225-256.

Unützer, J., Patrick, D. L., Simon, G., Grembowski, D., Walker, E., Rutter, C., & Katon, W. (1997). Depressive symptoms and the cost of health services in HMO patients age 65 years and older: A 4-year prospective study. *JAMA, 277*, 1618-1623.

Unützer, J., Patrick, D.L., Marmon, T., Simon, G.E., & Katon, W.J. (2002). Depressive symptoms and mortality in a prospective study of 2,558 older adults. *American Journal of Geriatric Psychiatry, 10*, 521-530.

van Eijk, J., Diederiks, J., Kempen, G., Honig, A., van der Meer, K., & Brenninkmeijer, W. (2004). Development and feasibility of a nurse administered strategy on depression in community-dwelling patients with a chronic physical disease. *Patient Education and Counseling, 34*, 87-94.

van Eijken, M., Wensing, M., de Konink, M., Vernooy, M., Zielhuis, G., Lagro, T. et al. (2004). Health education on self-management and seeking health care in older adults: A randomized trial. *Patient Education & Counseling, 55*(1), 48-54.

Virnig, B., Huang, Z., Lurie, N., Musgrave, D., McBean, A.M., & Dowd, B. (2004). Does Medicare managed care provide equal treatment for mental illness across races? *Archives of General Psychiatry, 61,* 201-205.

Wagner, E.H., Austin, B.T., & Von Korff, M. (1996). Organizing care for patients with chronic illness. *Milbank Quarterly, 7,* 511-44.

Wells, K. B., Sherbourne, C., Schoenbaum, M., Duan, N., Meredith, L., Unützer, J. et al. (2000). Impact of disseminating quality improvement programs for depression in managed primary care: A randomized controlled trial. *JAMA, 283,* 212-220.

Wells, K., Sherbourne, C., Schoenbaum, M., Ettner, S., Duan, N., Miranda, J. et al. (2004). Five-year impact of quality improvement for depression: Results of a group-level randomized controlled trial. *Archives of General Psychiatry, 61,* 378-86.

West, C.G., Reed, D.M., & Gildengorin, G.L. (1998). Can money buy happiness? Depressive symptoms in an affluent older population. *Journal of American Geriatrics Society, 46,* 49-57.

Wetherell, J.L., & Unützer, J. (2003). Adherence to treatment for geriatric depression and anxiety. *CNS Spectrums, 8(12 Suppl 3),* 48-59.

Whyte, E.M., Dew, M.A., Gildengers, A., Lenze, E.J., Bharucha, A., Mulsant, B.H., & Reynolds, C.F. (2004). Time course of response to antidepressants in late-life major depression: Therapeutic implications. *Drugs & Aging, 21,* 531-554.

Williams, J.W. Jr., Katon, W., Lin, E.H., Noel, P.H., Worchel, J., Cornell, J. et al. (2004). The effectiveness of depression care management on diabetes-related outcomes in older patients. *Annals of Internal Medicine, 140,* 1015-24.

Williams, J.W. Jr., Noel, P.H., Cordes, J.A., Ramirez, G., & Pignone, M. (2002). Is this patient clinically depressed? *JAMA, 287,* 1160-1170.

Williams, J.W., Barrett, J., Oxman, T., Frank, E., Katon, W., Sullivan, M. et al. (2000). Treatment of dysthymia and minor depression in primary care: A randomized controlled trial in older adults. *JAMA, 284,* 1519-1526.

Williams, J.W., Rost, K., Dietrich, A.J., Ciotti, M.C., Zyzanski, S.J., & Cornell, J. (1999). Primary care physicians' approach to depressive disorders: Effects of physician specialty and practice structure. *Archives of Family Medicine, 8,* 58-67.

Williams, M.L., & Payne, S. A. (2003). A qualitative study of clinical nurse specialists' views on depression in palliative care patients. *Palliative Medicine, 17,* 334-338.

Barriers and Facilitators to Replicating an Evidence-Based Palliative Care Model

E. Maxwell Davis, PhD Candidate
Paula Jamison, MA Candidate
Richard Brumley, MD
Susan Enguídanos, PhD, MPH

SUMMARY. Recognition of the difficulties involved in replicating evidence-based interventions is well documented in the literature within the medical field. Promising research findings are often not translated into practice, and if they are, there is a significant time gap between study conclusion and practice adoption. The purpose of this article is to describe the barriers and facilitators encountered by two managed care organizations while replicating an evidence-based end of life in-home palliative care model. Using Diffusion of Innovation Theory as a theoretical framework, results from focus groups and interviews with the project's clinical, administrative and research teams are presented and recommendations made for improving translational efforts. The process of replicating the end of life in-home palliative care model clearly illustrated the key elements required for successfully diffusing innovation. These key elements include marketing and communication, leadership, organizational support and training and mentorship. This qualitative

---

Address correspondence to: Susan Enguídanos, PhD, MPH, 732 Mott Street, Suite 150, San Fernando, CA 91340.

[Haworth co-indexing entry note]: "Barriers and Facilitators to Replicating an Evidence-Based Palliative Care Model." Davis, E. Maxwell et al. Co-published simultaneously in *Home Health Care Services Quarterly* (The Haworth Press, Inc.) Vol. 25, No. 1/2, 2006, pp. 149-165; and: *Evidence-Based Interventions for Community Dwelling Older Adults* (ed: Susan M. Enguídanos) The Haworth Press, Inc., 2006, pp. 149-165. Single or multiple copies of this article are available for a fee from The Haworth Document Delivery Service [1-800-HAWORTH, 9:00 a.m. - 5:00 p.m. (EST). E-mail address: docdelivery@haworthpress.com].

149

process study provides clear, real world perspectives of the myriad of challenges encountered in replicating an evidence-based project. *[Article copies available for a fee from The Haworth Document Delivery Service: 1-800-HAWORTH. E-mail address: <docdelivery@haworthpress.com> Website: <http://www.HaworthPress.com> © 2006 by The Haworth Press, Inc. All rights reserved.]*

KEYWORDS. Translational research, evidence-based practice, replication, end-of-life care, palliative care, diffusion theory, qualitative research, process study

INTRODUCTION

Recognition of the difficulties involved in replicating evidence-based interventions is well documented in the literature within the medical field. According to the Agency for Healthcare Research and Quality, the translation of research findings into clinical practice remains one of the largest hurdles to improving the quality, efficiency, effectiveness and cost-effectiveness of health care (AHRQ, 1999). Promising research findings are often not translated into practice, and if they are, there is a significant time gap between study conclusion and practice adoption. This may be due, in part, to the complexity of the research design and lack of transferability of the model into non-research settings. In addition, benefits of a research study may be diminished when translated into real-world practice settings (Gill, 2005; Glasgow, 2003). RE-AIM (Reach, Effectiveness, Adoption, Implementation, and Maintenance) describes key elements researchers need to embrace in designing an intervention that can be translated into practice (Glasgow, 2003). Studies that assess the reach, effectiveness, adoption, implementation, and maintenance from inception of the design have a greater ability to readily translate their findings into practice.

Translation of research to practice is slow, averaging about two decades to move from research to application (AHRQ, 1999; Eddy, 2005). Several studies have documented the significant time lapse that occurs in incorporating evidence-based knowledge into practice, which has occurred consistently throughout the history of modern medicine (Eddy, 2005). Given a robust study design and valid findings, there remain several obstacles in promoting the application of research to practice. According to Mullen (2004), several organizational and environmental supports need to be in place to buttress the use of evidence based practices. In addition, sufficient training must be available to adequately prepare clinicians to engage in the new practices.

The purpose of this article is to describe the barriers and facilitators encountered by two managed care organizations while replicating an evidence-based end of life in-home palliative care model. Using Diffusion of Innovation Theory as a theoretical framework, results from focus groups and interviews with the project's clinical, administrative and research teams will be presented and recommendations will be made for improving translational efforts. This article is intended to provide a review of both the underlying themes and the concrete reflections and suggestions that emerged from this process. In addition, these qualitative findings will provide information for others preparing to replicate evidence-based programs on avoiding and overcoming unexpected obstacles. This information is seen as critical to national efforts to disseminate responsive, best practice research, into the discourse around implementing evidence-based practice.

THEORETICAL FRAMEWORK

Berwick (2003) and the California HealthCare Foundation have suggested using Rogers' Diffusion of Innovation Theory (1995) as a theoretical framework to analyze the application of changing health care practices. This theory suggests that the rate of adoption of an innovation is influenced by several factors, namely, the perception of the innovation, characteristics of the people who adopt them, and contextual factors, such as communication, leadership, management, and incentives.

According to Rogers' Diffusion of Innovation Theory (1995), perception of the innovation involves five characteristics: relative advantage, compatibility, complexity, trialability and observability of the innovation. These factors figure significantly in predicting the rate of diffusion. Relative advantage is the degree to which an innovation is perceived to be better than the idea it replaces (Rogers, 1995), thus it is defined in terms of benefits and costs to the adopter. This may include factors such as improved benefit of the innovations for patients and reduced time or labor for the adopters. Compatibility is defined by how closely an innovation fits in with existing values and culture, past experiences, and the needs of adopters. Trialability addresses the degree to which an innovation may be tried out prior to full adoption, while complexity speaks to the difficulty of understanding and using the innovation. Complex interventions that are difficult to understand and implement are less likely to be adopted. Observability is the degree to which innovations provide readily observable positive results (Rogers, 1995). Those with clear positive results are more likely to be implemented.

Characteristics of the people who adopt innovations are also important factors associated with the diffusion process. Research has determined that not all individuals adopt innovations at the same rate and that an individual's personality and characteristics can determine how willing they are to adopt an innovation. Rogers (1995) has identified five categories of adopters that include: Innovators, Early Adopters, Early Majority, Late Majority, and Laggards. Innovators (about 2.5% of adopters) represent the fastest adopting group and generally are risk takers and leaders. These are followed by early adopters (about 13.5% of adopters) who are distinguished as opinion makers and have strong social connections that facilitate the spread of adoption to early majority who closely watch the actions of the early adopters. The early majority (34% of adopters) rely on their personal connections and knowledge. They serve as a link between early and late adopters and represent the point at which the innovation begins to take strong hold. The late majority (34%) are generally conservative and skeptical about new innovations. They observe the early majority for proof that the innovation works before they are persuaded to adopt. The Laggards (16%) are the last group to adopt. They generally do not like change and are unlikely to take risks and would prefer to stick to current methods.

Finally, Berwick (2003) describes contextual factors as the third cluster of influences on diffusion. These factors pertain to the managerial factors within the organization that facilitate or impede the adoption process. Organizations that encourage and support innovation will have improved rates of adoption. Additionally, organizations must have infrastructure to support the innovation. Leadership plays a critical role in diffusion of innovation process. Leaders that understand the need for innovation and that have a positive attitude toward change will foster innovation. Other organizational factors include complexity, interconnectedness, size and organizational slack. Communication is also a key factor in supporting and promoting innovation. Communication is the primary mechanism of diffusing information and is used at every stage of diffusion beginning at creating awareness, to transferring knowledge to changing attitudes through sharing knowledge.

BACKGROUND

In April 2001, funds were granted to conduct a replication project of an innovative program of palliative end of life care within two disparate managed care medical centers. The In-home Palliative Care Program (IPCP) is an interdisciplinary home-based model of care designed to provide treatment with the primary goals of enhancing comfort and improving quality of care in a patient's last year of life. The IPCP uses an interdisciplinary team approach, with the central care team composed of the patient and family, physician, nurse, and social worker, all with expertise in symptom management and biopsychosocial interventions. A nonequivalent comparison group study of the IPCP was conducted at Kaiser Permanente (KP) in Southern California. Findings from this study indicated that terminally ill persons enrolled in the IPCP cost 45% less than patients enrolled in traditional care and were more satisfied than those in traditional care at 60 days following enrollment (Brumley, Enguídanos, & Cherin, 2003).

The replication process entailed a very thorough and lengthy orientation process that began with a visit from the replication site representatives to the original program location (home site) for a general overview of palliative care. Representatives from the replication sites were presented with a review of end-of-life care topics, including pain and symptom control and advanced care planning. In addition, day-to-day operations of running a palliative care program were discussed including clinical and administrative issues. Modeling and observation were key elements of the training curriculum. Replication site team members observed the home site's intake and discharge procedures, attended in-home palliative care patient visits along with a multi-disciplinary staff, reviewed documentation requirements and protocols, and participated in a case conference meeting.

In June of 2001, members of the home site's palliative care team then visited the two replication sites in order to conduct on-site training sessions. Prospective clinical staff including physicians, registered nurses, social workers, chaplains, and volunteers was invited to participate. Similar to the training sessions that took place at the home site, on-site trainings at replication sites consisted of an overview of the program from intake to discharge or transition into other programs such as hospice. During this overview, process adaptations were discussed based upon the organizational variations present at each replication site. Home site training facilitators provided a general review of end-of-life care, presented cases for management, and reviewed quality indicators.

In addition, strategies for marketing the new program were discussed in order to generate referrals to the newly developed palliative care programs. These strategies included the development of brochures, email newsletters to be distributed monthly to clinical staff, and delivery of a presentation to be given to potential referring physicians by replication site physician leaders.

Significant differences exist between the two replication sites in regards to their organizational structures and the populations served, which impacted the replication process and practice of palliative care at each site. One site provides home health and hospice services by a contracted agency as opposed to having these services in-house. In addition, the ethnic background of the majority of their patients is primarily Caucasian. Conversely, the other replication site has its own hospital-based, home health agency, with hospice services provided externally by contracted agencies. In addition, the ethnic background of this replication site's population was predominantly Asian/Pacific Islanders. These varying organizational structures and patient demographics between sites were factors that had a significant impact on the process of replicating the palliative care model.

METHODS

Approximately 18 months after the initiation of the Palliative Care study within the two managed care sites, a qualitative process study was undertaken to identify institutional and programmatic barriers and facilitators experienced during the replication of the model. Toward this end, the evaluator conducted three focus groups with care team members who were directly involved with the implementation of the IPCP at each site. The dialogue in these groups focused on care team members' reflections on the process of implementing such a program, their impressions of the training and ongoing support that they received from the home site during the implementation process, and their suggestions for replication of the model at future sites.

The evaluator conducted 11 individual interviews with oncologists, pulmonologists and internal medicine physicians. Specific efforts were taken to ensure inclusion of physicians and specialists making both low and high volumes of referrals to the program. These open-ended, structured interviews focused on eliciting physician perceptions as to the structural and experiential barriers and facilitators to the referral process and their suggestions for improving that process.

Finally, individual interviews were conducted with the two administrators at the home site who oversaw the implementation of the IPCP program at both replication sites. These conversations focused on the administrators' reflections on the process of implementing the program at each site and on their impressions of where their efforts struggled and succeeded in this process. They also offered ideas about modifications to be made in future replication efforts.

RESULTS

Using the Diffusion of Innovations model, the process of implementing the IPCP program at each site can be examined in terms of identified facilitators of and barriers to the process of replication and dissemination.

Perceptions of the Innovation: Facilitators and Barriers of the Replication Process

Increasing Awareness

In order to facilitate diffusion of innovation, it was necessary to devise a marketing strategy that demonstrated the value of palliative care for the physicians, patients and the organization in general. Individuals from one site expressed the belief that both staff (administrators and referring physicians) and patient families were less than open to the introduction of a new program and to an innovation in ways of providing care. They attribute this, at least in part, to the challenge of introducing new practices into a somewhat isolated community wherein exposure to innovation is infrequent and not often positively reinforced. One team member commented that "we have a sense of isolation in [our community]. . . Despite telephones and email, we sort of continue to do things the same way because new blood is seldom introduced." As one high-referring physician asserted, the biggest determinant of whether or not a doctor refers to a program like this is "how interested that doctor is in getting his or her patients involved in that program."

The successful dissemination of the IPCP program at each site consisted of developing buy-in among the physicians from whom patient referrals were needed in order to populate the program. Because of this, an early goal of the program implementation process was to communicate to referring physicians the worth, effectiveness, and benefits of palliative care to their patients and how the model complemented the care that they provide. In addition, the marketing strategy included a detailed explanation regarding the value of conducting a study to test the effectiveness of the innovation. These messages were disseminated both through active marketing of the palliative care program prior to its inception and through ongoing presentations and feedback provided to all physicians throughout the implementation process. In addition, palliative care team members provided regular and rapid feedback to referring physicians regarding each individual patient referred and accepted into the program.

These efforts appear to have been successful in developing the perception among physicians that the IPCP program was a good one and that the care provided appropriately matched patient needs and wishes. These messages seem to have been a central facilitator of the referral process and thus the dissemination of this innovation. Almost all high-referring physicians, as well as some low-referring internal medicine physicians, commented during interviews that they saw the program as a great one and that they viewed the availability of home care and the option for patients to continue treatment as major assets of the program. A few physicians also articulated their belief that palliative care is desirable because it is cost effective. These physicians indicated that awareness of these features made them more likely to refer patients. One referring physician even commented that he "[sees] this program as the kind of program [he'd] want to be in at the end of his life."

Ensuring Clarity

Although providing a marketing protocol emphasizing the positive aspects of a program is imperative, it is also necessary to assure adequate education regarding the proposed innovative program is provided. The IPCP program required that physicians from several specialties refer to the program; as a result, barriers in referring patients arose due to a lack of clarity about the program in terms of knowledge and understanding of its goals and boundaries. This presented challenges to its dissemination both initially and over the life of the dissemination process of the project. Some clinicians felt that despite the initial training in palliative care and ongoing support encouraging continued referral of patient,

> one thing that was not made explicit was exactly what palliative care was. . . We have all, as individuals, interpreted that differently and that has caused a lot of trouble in our implementation, in terms

of mixed messages to families, to doctors, to other team members, etc.

The ongoing struggle to secure patient referrals at each of the program sites was largely related to referring physicians' lack of clarity regarding the program and the process associated with enrolling a patient. In explaining low referral practices, physicians referenced several perceptions that inhibited them, including misperceptions about the nature of service eligibility criteria. Several listed entirely different perceived criteria for eligibility, indicating an overall lack of clarity about the actual criteria. Interviews with referring physicians revealed that by far the most significant barrier to their making referrals to the program was the perception that referring a patient meant losing control of that patient's care and/or being sidelined during decision-making processes. One high-referring physician asserted that referring doctors were more likely to be comfortable with referring patients to the program if they "understand that they will continue to be a part of the patient care team and have input into patient care." He suggested that in order to help physicians feel more at ease with this, the program must engage in ongoing publicity and do a better job of "selling the teamwork concept" and "stressing that care is managed as a team." Clearly communicating the program requirements, goals, and objectives is critical to assuring the successful adoption of an innovation.

Characteristics of Adopters

Certain characteristics were present among the individuals who eventually became stewards of the ICPC implementation, dissemination at the replication sites and members of its core care teams. These site leaders were innovators, since before the replication study was initiated, they had already begun a "grassroots effort" to bring palliative care to their site. They note, though, that they did not know how to accomplish that task with regard to issues like staffing, budgeting and utilizing organizational relationships. Thus, they recognized the need to integrate knowledge from other sources into the program implementation process and to seek dialogue with their administrative officers about program needs and outcomes. Another essential characteristic of these innovators was the commitment to improving end of life care. This trait was present in the majority of physicians and care team members at both replication sites, who observed that they entered the pilot project with the belief that palliative care work is special and valuable.

Certain key characteristics also seem to describe those physicians who embraced the IPCP program by referring patients to the program early and often. Interviews with physicians revealed patterns in their referring experiences and behaviors that cluster by program site, medical specialty and level of referrals. For instance, a number of high-referring physicians indicated that they see a disproportionate number of very sick, older and/or dying patients and therefore may be more comfortable with the idea of palliative care. High-referring physicians also expressed a focus on the overall welfare of dying patients rather than on specialty-specific protocols and regimens. Finally, those physicians who made high volumes of referrals to the IPCP program seemed to have fewer "turf" issues around control over patient care than those who did not. One of these physicians noted this issue and expressed with regret that his colleagues who most fear the loss of control over patient care simply did not make referrals to the program and thus were never able to realize that their fears were unfounded.

Finally, physicians who were late adopters or laggards in adopting the IPCP program by not making high levels of referrals seem to share some key characteristics as well. In interviews, several low-referring physicians discussed their wish to retain complete control over patient care issues as a barrier to referring to the palliative care program. One low-referring physician indicates that doctors "generally don't accurately communicate with patients and families what the patient's prognosis is as they are hesitant to say 'you may not be around in 6 months' and will just keep going on with treatment instead." Another physician indicated that some of her patients have felt abandoned by her after being referred, as she is no longer as involved with them once they are accepted into the program, and that this became a barrier for her.

Contextual Factors

A number of positive contextual factors around leadership, management and communication style helped to buttress the dissemination of this program's innovations.

Leadership

One of the key elements observed early on by the home site staff was the need for strong physician leadership to the project. Specifically, sites with physician leaders that were well established, respected by their staff, peers and administrations, were more successful in their program implementation. The sharing of the leadership role was also key in ensuring continuity of the program in the absence of a physician leader. Team members pointed out that when even one physician went on vacation or left to attend a training seminar, this created a major deficiency for the program.

As present at the replication sites, it is necessary that the program leaders share a deep philosophical and practical commitment to the palliative care model and to providing superior patient care prior in their medical practice. Interviews reveal their shared passion for providing palliative care and their shared belief that such work is special and valuable. This consistency of values among care teams allowed them to establish trust and build collaborative, as well as create reciprocal relationships among themselves, administration and patients at each of the replication sites. This in turn facilitated the IPCP program's early functioning at each site. Care team members saw this capacity for team building as inherent to the nature of the palliative care model and as manifested by their mutual support and reinforcement of program achievements and relationships.

In general, care team members also saw themselves as special in certain ways and assert that disseminating a program like this one requires finding key players of a certain temperament. In concrete terms, these staff members were willing to devote far more hours to work on the IPCP program than they were required to over the course of the implementation period. They feel strongly that it is critical to secure committed, invested care providers like themselves, arguing that "you can't just have someone who's showing up for a paycheck" doing this kind of work. Some acknowledge, however, that their initial level of investment in the program (i.e., taking call 24/7 for months at a time) proved to be draining and ultimately un-sustainable. In addition, the home site program administrators who were responsible for securing funding for this program, managing it, conducting all training and providing all ongoing support for the care teams spent far more time working on these goals than they were "officially" slated to and felt that this time was necessary in order to achieve the goals of the program.

Administration/Management

One of the core areas influencing diffusion of the model was in gathering and maintaining upper level administrative support for staff resources. Replication site care team members consistently perceived a conflict between their core values about the IPCP program's purpose and worth and those of some of the organization's administrators. Thus, an important role of the home site was providing support in facing these challenges. This was done initially through meetings and presentation of data from the original study and also later by providing ongoing data and discussion as needed. In addition, many of home site's experiences with getting this project off the ground mirror those of the care teams, in terms of having to deal with issues around insufficient resource allocation, unmet needs and unanticipated problems and instabilities. Therefore the care team members' needs were being heard and understood by people in a position of relative power who could both empathize with their struggles and advocate for their needs.

The most common contextual problems at both sites involved insufficient resource allocation and a general lack of knowledge of and facility with staffing, budgetary issues and administrative and systemic processes on the part of care team leaders. In retrospect, both care team members and program administrators viewed the funding plan for the project as inadequate, both in terms of dollars and time allocated. They continue to express dismay at the degree to which the possibilities for a program like this one are dictated by financial versus patient care issues. One team member noted that

> to sell this to the organization, part of what you have to sell is how it needs to be done: how slowly it needs to start, what kinds of resources need to be committed, what needs to be done for team building, because trust us, it will pay off down the road. It will run smoothly and all of these things that contribute to poor patient management will be alleviated. That's something that they should take advantage of if they're going to replicate this kind of model.

Another resource need identified was staffing. Staffing, in terms of the staff time allocated for work on this project, remained a major issue at both the home site (to provide guidance, supervision and training) and replication sites throughout the program implementation process. Both care teams note that fluctuations in staffing needs sometimes created chaotic circumstances wherein outside staff had to be pulled in to meet unanticipated care needs, with uneven results. They were also frustrated by the fact that their team composition kept changing and that this sometimes meant working with clinicians who had no experience providing end-of-life care.

Further, both proximity of location from the home site and the substantial organization structural variation from the home site affected

diffusion efforts and the level of training required. Home site administrators note that the lack of proximity between the home site and program replication sites presented some challenges in terms of the
mentorship and ongoing training and support of team members and contributed to the dearth of experiential components in both the initial training and ongoing support efforts. Organization structural variation from
the home site included a patient population that was largely culturally
different from home site and the need to partner with outside care agencies to conduct the IPCP. The partner agency was unstable, resulting in
complex, conflicted relationships, organizational divisions and geographic distance between care team members. They describe feeling
battle weary in the wake of a program implementation process that has
been fraught with scattered management styles and intense struggles,
both within the organization and between their organization and their
partner agency and believe that all of these factors have complicated
their dissemination process.

Training

Training, mentoring, and ongoing support proved to be the most critical aspect of the replication process. The in-person training and ongoing
support efforts stand out as especially important among both home and
replication site staff. Members of both teams identify all training efforts
as critical to their learning processes. They also see the most useful and
meaningful training and support forums being interactive activities like
conference calls, face-to-face meetings and site visits.

Both replication teams report receiving both concrete/practical and
motivational/emotional support from the home site throughout the implementation process. They also identify the home site's provision of
ongoing mentorship and consistent and frequent validation regarding
ongoing successes and milestones as essential.

Neither the on-site staff nor the home site administrators anticipated
that more training time was needed to ensure that all care team members
fully grasped the myriad of issues involved in palliative care and to prepare care team members to handle administrative issues such as cost
management, staffing decisions and administrative interactions. In addition, the home site administrators did not anticipate the degree to
which both care teams wanted and needed face-to-face contact for training and support. One home site administrator noted, "we overestimated
the level of comfort and training around palliative care provision among
the clinicians involved at both sites; we thought they had more clinical

experience, and it turned out that we overestimated both." Members of both replication teams recognize in retrospect that they were not able to articulate what kinds of support they needed at key moments, largely because they were not yet far enough along in their learning processes to appropriately identify their own needs. They reflect on this by noting that "in retrospect we should have called and told [home site administrator] that we needed him again" when questions and problems first arose.

Recommendations

The process of replicating the IPCP model clearly illustrated the key elements required for successfully diffusing innovation. Specifically the key elements include:

Marketing & Communication. Maintaining open and consistent communication between sites for clinical and administrative consultation via telephone and face to face is needed to ensure continuity of replication and fidelity to the original model. In addition, to gather and maintain organizational support from both administrators and physicians, regular communication and program promotion activities are required.

Leadership. Identifying physician leaders that are well established, respected by their staff, peers and administrations, and have the authority to implement clinical policies. Leadership should not be relegated to one individual; program leadership should be shared by two or more physicians so that the program is not jeopardized by the absence of one leader.

Organizational/Administrative Support. Lack of or insufficient levels of administrative support can prove to be detrimental to replication efforts. Ensure sufficient funding and resources (staffing and support) are allocated to the project before initiating the program. Obtain administrative commitment to the project for the entire project period. Be sure to allocate sufficient resources to include time needed to market the program to physicians and leaders. Replication site physician leaders should obtain written commitment from administration (both locally and regionally) in order to reduce threats to the program should local leadership change.

Training & Mentorship. Thorough training and ongoing mentorship and support are core components in establishing and maintaining fidelity to the original program model. Establish a comprehensive training schedule with ongoing mentoring and training opportunities for all types of staff involved with the program, including the inevitable new hires replacing previously trained staff. Training sessions should include experiential methods such as role-playing and reviewing case studies with palliative care staff, provided both on-site and via distance. Develop explicit clinical guidelines detailing the techniques and activities used with actual patient experiences of staff in order to share with replication clinical teams.

CONCLUSION

This qualitative process study provides clear, real world perspectives of the myriad of challenges encountered in replicating an evidence-based project. It also illuminates the important factors that must be considered and addressed when diffusing innovation within health care settings. The findings discussed in this paper are consistent with several other studies' experience conducting translational research.

Introducing innovation requires change in current practice standards organizationally and individually, which is always difficult to institute. Kilbourne et al. (2004) found that when translating an evidence-based, cost effective model of depression management into the primary care setting, changing practice proved to be extremely difficult due to organizational, financial and individual barriers. Changing individual behavior is a daunting task even when only one clinical practice guideline is altered. For example, despite a plethora of evidence published regarding the most appropriate treatment for high blood pressure, recent research studies suggest that physicians are not prescribing the appropriate medications for most of their hypertensive patients (Holmes, Shevrin, Goldman, & Share, 2004). This is primarily attributed to a lack of effective dissemination of practice guidelines to physicians and patients.

Nananda Col (2005) identified the primary impediments of disseminating evidence-based models into clinical practice. Some of these barriers include difficulty in effectively communicating research findings into terminology familiar to clinicians and appropriately targeting clinicians for dissemination of the model. Communicating effectively and establishing buy in from clinical staff and organizational leadership are key elements needed to ensure successful replication of an evidence-based model. This was not only a key finding from the IPCP project but within other research studies as well. Although translating evidence-based research into practice is complicated, it is a critical task that must be conducted more frequently in order to improve the efficacy and quality of clinical practice.

The individuals involved in the IPCP replication project described feeling both highly energized by their ideals and very much over-whelmed by the administrative realities of the organization. They noted that replicating this model forced them to acquire new non-clinical skills, such as an understanding of the administrative perspective and the importance of social capital in an undertaking like this one and that this context of growth has furthered their appreciation of what these types of innovations require from all players. Further, all IPCP partici-pants appear to have gradually developed the recognition that dissemi-nation of this type of innovation requires changing not only their thoughts and behaviors but those of others as well.

Replication site staff describe providing care through the IPCP pro-gram as demanding but rewarding, involving both extreme frustration and deep satisfaction. They discuss the process of changing practice it-self as a challenging one and describe many of their struggles and solu-tions in relation to their personal evolution and growth around that process. Both replication teams believe that participation in the pallia-tive care program has been valuable to them as practitioners and profes-sionals as well as to the patients for whom they have provided care. One care team member comments on this by saying "what we're doing is amazing. You can hear it in the patients' voices, you can see it in the in-dividual outcomes, and we could do it even better. It's some of the most wonderful and the most painful work all of us have ever done."

REFERENCES

AHRQ. (1999). *Translating Research into Practice II*. Retrieved December 16, 1999, from *http://grants.nih.gov/grants/guide/rfa-files/RFA-HS-00-008.html*

Berwick, D. M. (2003). Disseminating innovations in health care. *Jama, 289*(15), 1969-1975.

Brumley, R. D., Enguidanos, S., & Cherin, D. (2003). Effectiveness of a Home-Based Palliative Care Program for End-of-Life. *Journal of Palliative Medicine, 6*(5), 715-724.

Col, N. F. (2005). Challenges in translating research into practice. *J Womens Health (Larchmt), 14*(1), 87-95.

Eddy, D. M. (2005). Evidence-based medicine: A unified approach. *Health Aff (Millwood), 24*(1), 9-17.

Gill, T. M. (2005). Education, prevention, and the translation of research into practice. *J Am Geriatr Soc, 53*(4), 724-726.

Glasgow, R. E. (2003). Translating research to practice: Lessons learned, areas for im-provement, and future directions. *Diabetes Care, 26*(8), 2451-2456.

Holmes, J. S., Shevrin, M., Goldman, B., & Share, D. (2004). Translating research into practice: Are physicians following evidence-based guidelines in the treatment of hypertension? *Med Care Res Rev, 61*(4), 453-473.

Kilbourne, A. M., Schulberg, H. C., Post, E. P., Rollman, B. L., Belnap, B. H., & Pincus, H. A. (2004). Translating evidence-based depression management services to community-based primary care practices. *Milbank Q, 82*(4), 631-659.

Mullen, R. (2004). Evidence for whom?: ASHA's National Outcomes Measurement System. *J Commun Disord, 37*(5), 413-417.

Rogers, E. (1995). *Diffusion of Innovations* (Fourth Edition ed.). New York: The Free Press.

Index

BOOK ORDER FORM!

Order a copy of this book with this form or online at:
http://www.HaworthPress.com/store/product.asp?sku= 5858

Evidence-Based Interventions
for Community Dwelling Older Adults

_____ in softbound at $19.95 ISBN-13: 978-0-7890-3284-3 / ISBN-10: 0-7890-3284-8.
_____ in hardbound at $36.95 ISBN-13: 978-0-7890-3283-6 / ISBN-10: 0-7890-3283-X.

COST OF BOOKS _____

POSTAGE & HANDLING _____
US: $4.00 for first book & $1.50
for each additional book
Outside US: $5.00 for first book
& $2.00 for each additional book.

SUBTOTAL _____

In Canada: add 7% GST. _____

STATE TAX _____
CA, IL, IN, MN, NJ, NY, OH, PA & SD residents
please add appropriate local sales tax.

FINAL TOTAL _____

If paying in Canadian funds, convert
using the current exchange rate,
UNESCO coupons welcome.

❑ **BILL ME LATER:**
Bill-me option is good on US/Canada/
Mexico orders only; not good to jobbers,
wholesalers, or subscription agencies.

❑ **Signature** _____

❑ **Payment Enclosed: $**_____

❑ **PLEASE CHARGE TO MY CREDIT CARD:**

❑ Visa ❑ MasterCard ❑ AmEx ❑ Discover
❑ Diner's Club ❑ Eurocard ❑ JCB

Account #_____

Exp Date_____

Signature_____
(Prices in US dollars and subject to change without notice.)

PLEASE PRINT ALL INFORMATION OR ATTACH YOUR BUSINESS CARD

Name

Address

City   State/Province   Zip/Postal Code

Country   Tel

Fax   E-Mail

May we use your e-mail address for confirmations and other types of information? ❑Yes ❑No We appreciate receiving
your e-mail address. Haworth would like to e-mail special discount offers to you, as a preferred customer.
We will never share, rent, or exchange your e-mail address. We regard such actions as an invasion of your privacy.

Order from your **local bookstore** or directly from
The Haworth Press, Inc. 10 Alice Street, Binghamton, New York 13904-1580 • USA
Call our toll-free number (1-800-429-6784) / Outside US/Canada: (607) 722-5857
Fax: 1-800-895-0582 / Outside US/Canada: (607) 771-0012
E-mail your order to us: orders@HaworthPress.com

For orders outside US and Canada, you may wish to order through your local
sales representative, distributor, or bookseller.
For information, see http://HaworthPress.com/distributors

(Discounts are available for individual orders in US and Canada only, not booksellers/distributors.)

The Haworth Press Inc.

Please photocopy this form for your personal use.
www.HaworthPress.com

BOF06